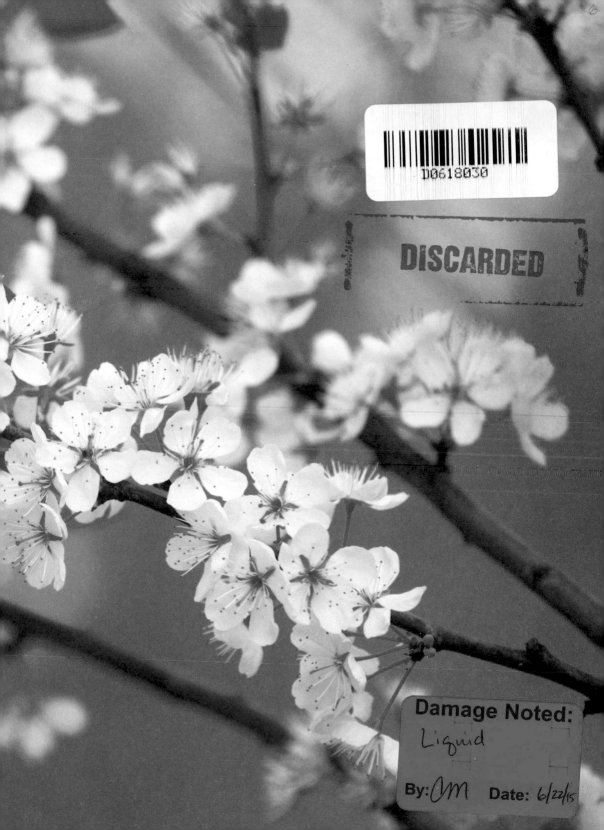

FERTILITY & CONCEPTION

the natural way

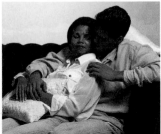

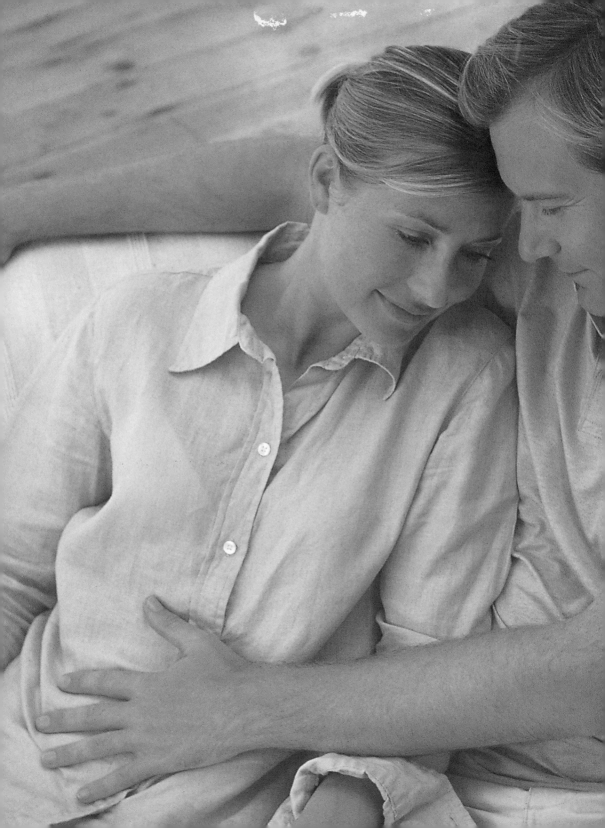

FERTILITY & CONCEPTION
the natural way

boost your chances of getting pregnant
and prepare for a successful birth and a
healthy baby using natural therapies,
diet and simple exercise regimes

ANNE CHARLISH
AND KIM DAVIES

LORENZ BOOKS

This edition is published by Lorenz Books, an imprint of Anness Publishing Ltd,
Blaby Road, Wigston, Leicestershire LE18 4SE; info@anness.com

www.lorenzbooks.com; www.annesspublishing.com

If you like the images in this book and would like to investigate using them for publishing, promotions
or advertising, please visit our website www.practicalpictures.com for more information.

Publisher: Joanna Lorenz
Editorial Director: Helen Sudell
Project Editor: Ann Kay
Copy Editor: Kim Davies
Designer: Lisa Tai
Jacket design: Adelle Morris
Special Photography: Alistair Hughes
Illustrations: Sam Elmhurst
Production: Wanda Burrows, Claire Rae

© Anness Publishing Ltd 2012

A CIP catalogue record for this book is available from the British Library.

Publisher's Note
The information in this book and the opinions of the authors should not be regarded as a substitute for attention
from a qualified health professional. If you are suffering from any medical complaint, or are worried about any
aspect of your health, you must get a medical opinion. Always seek advice before starting any exercise programme,
whether you are pregnant or not, but especially during pregnancy. The publishers can take no responsibility for any
kind of injury or illness resulting from the advice given or the exercises and routines demonstrated in this book.
At the time of writing, the authors had made every effort, as far as they were able, to ensure that the information
in this book was accurate, up to date and in accordance with current practices and guidelines.

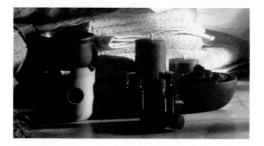

contents

Introduction

" Once you have decided to embark upon this incredible journey, then a whole new world opens up to you. "

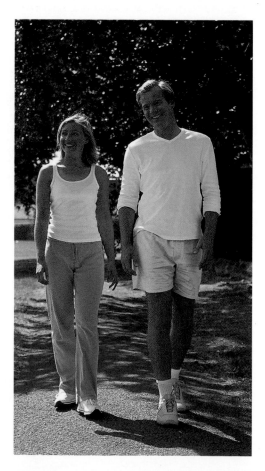

The desire to conceive is one of the most basic and powerful of human instincts, shared with all the living things on our planet. Once you have decided to embark upon this incredible journey, then a whole new world opens up to you. The key at this time is to gather as much information as possible, and to maintain optimum physical well-being and a healthy mental outlook.

Preparing properly for pregnancy is vital and this book takes an evenly balanced, two-handed approach. On the one hand, it gives the prospective mother and father all the scientific facts they need to know about the miracle of conceiving a baby. It outlines thoroughly all the factors that can affect pregnancy, such as age and specific medical problems, and explains clearly all the medical tests and solutions that are available.

On the other hand, this book also places a very strong emphasis on the importance of following a well-tailored natural preconception programme, looking at how you can support your goal through

Keeping yourselves as fit and active as possible is a vital part of any preconceptual care programme. Get out and walk instead of taking numerous trips in the car.

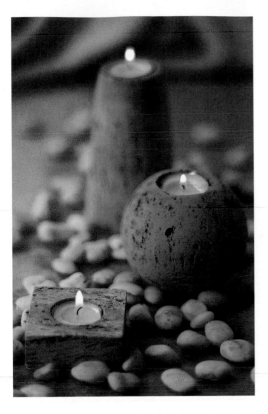

All kinds of holistic therapies can assist women through every stage of conception, and then of pregnancy – even if it is simply burning aromatic candles to create a calm and serene atmosphere.

TAKE CARE

This book has been written with the aim of helping women who are trying to conceive. However, it is very important to remember that no book can be a substitute for getting advice about your own specific medical circumstances. For this reason, all of the suggestions contained in this book should only be followed under the informed guidance of your doctor and a properly qualified complementary practitioner.

If you are at all worried by any symptom you may have, suffer from a specific medical complaint, or are unsure about whether or not a natural therapy is safe, do not hesitate to consult your family doctor.

At any point while attempting to conceive, you could already be pregnant. Seek immediate medical help if you experience any of the following symptoms:

- Vaginal bleeding other than light spotting (or menstruation).
- Severe abdominal pain, especially if you are also bleeding vaginally.
- Continuous and severe headache, with or without blurred vision and with or without swelling of the hands and ankles.
- Excessive vomiting in which you cannot keep down any food or liquid, even water. Telephone your family doctor promptly if you notice the following:
- A temperature of 38.5°C (101°F) or more.
- Sudden swelling of the hands and ankles. If you also have blurred vision and/or severe headache as well as the swelling, you should call an ambulance.
- Urinating not only frequently (which is normal during pregnancy) but also with pain when you pass water, as this usually signifies some kind of infection.

improving diet and well-being, following the right kind of exercise regime and selecting what's right for you from a host of supportive complementary therapies – from yoga and homeopathy to meditation and herbalism. Complementary therapies can help you to boost your immune system, raise your energy levels and achieve a state of calm, and may also allow you to sit back and take stock of your life, to see where you may need to make adjustments and perhaps simplify your life.

This kind of preparation not only puts you in the best all-round shape to conceive a healthy baby, but also sets you up for your challenging new life as parents. Conceiving a baby is probably the most joyful event of your lives. Be sure that this is the right time for you and your partner and prepare as well as you can. You have everything to look forward to.

CHAPTER ONE
Preparing for conception

❝ Enjoy all the new things that you will be discovering about yourself. ❞

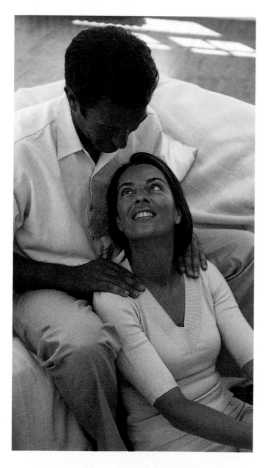

Having a child is a wonderful event, but of course it is also a life-changing one. The decision to try for a baby is one that no one else can make for you – only you know whether this is a course that you truly wish to embark on.

As you explore this exciting change in your life, consider both the emotional and practical issues. Think about the strength of the relationship with your partner, and discuss possible parenthood thoroughly with them. Weigh up your age, your current income and work prospects, your living arrangements and whether there is sufficient space for a baby. Ask yourself whether or not you really feel ready to become responsible for a new life. After all, a child will be with you for many years to come.

Find out as much as you can about pregnancy, labour, and being a parent. Talk to other parents, and spend time with people who have young children so that you get a real taste of just what it may be like.

If you have a partner, your relationship will need to be strong as you start along the road to parenthood. Many decisions lie ahead, which should be made together.

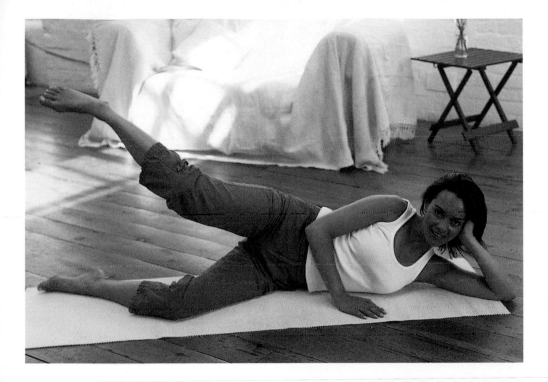

Choosing to have a child involves both instinct and reason. Don't worry if you have doubts, as no one can be totally certain of any choice that they make. We can only decide what feels right for us and then pursue our chosen goal in a positive spirit.

If you decide to go ahead, you will want to prepare as well as possible. You may need to improve your general health or fitness or lose or gain weight before trying to conceive. Look into ways of eating healthy, natural foods and find out about the wide choice of complementary therapies that will help to keep you in top mental and physical shape. Above all, enjoy all the new things that you will be discovering about yourself as well as the journey ahead of you.

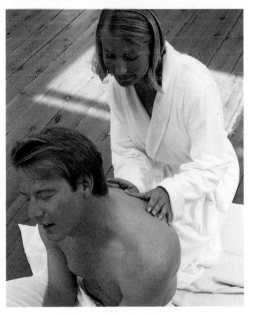

Top: Keep yourself in good physical shape, but avoid suddenly starting a tough routine that you have never tried before, and seek advice from your doctor first.

Help to strengthen your relationship, and keep stress at bay, by making time to enjoy relaxing and sensual pleasures such as a soothing massage.

Deciding to have a baby

Choosing to have a baby is without question the most momentous decision of your life. No other will have such far-reaching, and yet such potentially rewarding, implications over the years to come.

Some people feel an absolute certainty that they are ready to have a baby. Others feel more ambivalent about the effect that a child may have on their lifestyle or relationship. In addition, partners often feel differently about exactly when or if they want to become parents.

Discussing all the issues is essential. It is important that you ask yourself some searching questions before going ahead, and that you and your partner are honest about any hopes and fears that you have.

WHY YOU WANT TO HAVE A BABY
Talking about your reasons for wanting a baby can help you to pinpoint any assumptions that you have about the role a child will play in your life. For example, do you see a baby as something that will enhance an already happy life – or as a way of filling an emotional void? Are you hoping he or she will strengthen a loving partnership – or cement over the cracks in a rocky one?

It would not be wise to conceive a child in order to repair problems in your relationship or simply because you want to have someone to love. If there are tensions between you and your partner, having a baby will almost certainly exacerbate them – lack of sleep and having more to do at home soon cause tempers to fray.

Caring for a baby can be an isolating experience, especially if you do not have a loving partner to lean on. Many people bring up their children as lone parents – and do a wonderful job. Ideally, though, you will be in a committed, loving relationship that is strong enough to withstand the challenges of bringing up a child.

PROGRESSING TO PARENTHOOD
One of the most important things for you and your partner to consider is whether or not you feel ready to welcome another person into your relationship. Are you sufficiently certain of your feelings for one another to be able to care for a helpless and dependent baby?

Think, too, about whether your partner is the person you want to parent your child. Do you consider him or her to be sufficiently mature, kind, compassionate, intelligent, and sensitive to be your co-parent? As a hypothetical question, would you have liked your partner as a parent yourself? Try to imagine it just for a moment.

YOUR LIFESTYLE
Before trying to conceive, discuss how you see your lives adapting to a new child. Consider some of the practical issues. Is your home a suitable place for a child, for example, or will you have to move? Is one of you planning to stay at home with the baby for the first years? If so, is the other prepared to be sole breadwinner for a time?

If your career is important to you, think about whether you can take some time off without damaging your future prospects. Consider, too, how you will cope with both the costs of having a child and the likely reduction in your income as a result of working less or paying for childcare.

Take some time to think about how you see your lives in five or ten years' time. Is what you want in terms of

FERTILITY ISSUES TO CONSIDER
When considering whether or not this is the right time to try for a baby, you may need to consider biological factors. Most important of these is the age of the woman.

A woman's fertility decreases as she gets older, particularly after the age of 35. Fertility starts to decrease about ten years before a woman's periods stop, and most women start the menopause around 45–55 (though it can be much earlier). There is no way of knowing exactly when the menopause will start, so it is wise not to put off conceiving for too long, particularly if you are already in your thirties.

From a biological point of view, a woman is most likely to conceive between 20 and 25 years of age. If you delay having a child until later, be aware that you are more likely to experience delays in conception than younger women. However, age usually brings with it greater stability and maturity, which are vital factors where parenthood is concerned.

Many different factors may be involved in the timing of your pregnancy. If both you and your partner feel that you are ready to have a child together, then this is probably the right time for you to go ahead, irrespective of work, finances or any other concerns.

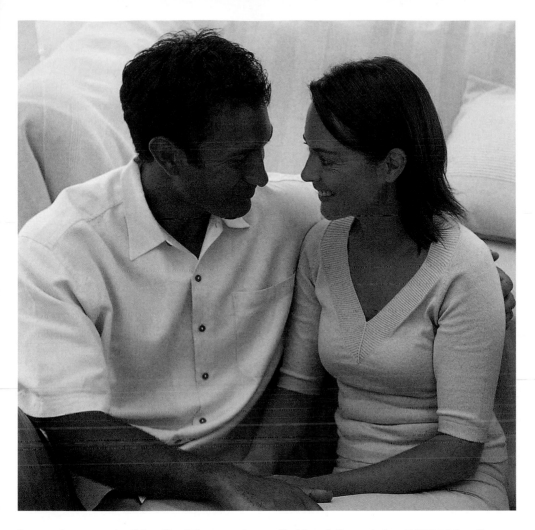

home and career compatible with what your partner wants? Are you agreed on how you see your future lives?

None of these issues is likely to be the deciding factor in whether or not you try to start a family. However, discussing them can help to build up a picture of how you and your partner feel about starting a family, and whether or not you need to make changes to your lifestyle first.

YOUR SUPPORT NETWORK

Family and close friends can be a vital support when you have a baby – particularly in the first few months when you are adjusting to your new lifestyle. It is a good idea to discuss with your partner the role that each of your families may play in helping you. Do you have supportive friends or relatives near to where you live at the moment? If not, would you consider moving?

Deciding whether, and when, to have a baby will probably be the biggest and most important event of your lives together – and the most exciting.

MAKING A DECISION

Ultimately, only you and your partner can know if this is the right time for you to try for a baby. Give yourselves plenty of time to make the decision, and listen carefully to what your inner voice tells you.

Listen just as carefully to what your partner says – and make sure that you hear what he or she actually says, rather than what you wish to hear. It is easy to imagine that your partner's aims are the same as yours, but this isn't always the case. Having a baby is a long-term commitment and both partners need to be sure that this is what they really want.

How conception happens

For pregnancy to occur, both the man's and the woman's reproductive system must be in good working order, the couple must make love at the right time of the woman's menstrual cycle, and her body must produce a complex chain of hormones in order to keep the pregnancy going.

When a man ejaculates during sexual intercourse, millions of sperm are released into the woman's vagina. They move up the vagina and through the cervix into the uterus, propelled both by the force of ejaculation and by moving their tails like tiny fish. From there, the sperm make their way to the Fallopian tubes. This process is like a frantic race, as only one sperm among the millions can fertilize the egg. The rest fall away before they reach the goal, or else arrive too late.

If sexual intercourse has taken place without contraception, some sperm may reach the Fallopian tube and a single one may fertilize the waiting egg. The fertilized egg then makes its way towards the woman's uterus (womb), where it attaches itself to the lining. Here, it develops first into a tiny embryo, then a fetus and, eventually, into a baby.

THE WOMAN'S REPRODUCTIVE SYSTEM

A woman's reproductive system lies within her pelvis, and consists of the ovaries, the Fallopian tubes, the uterus, the cervix, the vagina and the vulva.

Baby girls are born with all their eggs in place in the ovaries – about 2–3 million of them. The ovaries are dormant during childhood and start to function only as puberty and menstruation begins. From then, women of childbearing age release an egg every four weeks or so. This monthly timetable is called the ovulatory or menstrual cycle. About 400–500 eggs are released during a woman's childbearing years – before ovulation ceases at menopause, usually in the woman's forties or fifties.

At the beginning of the ovulatory cycle, a number of eggs begin to grow in the ovaries. After about 14 days, one egg is mature enough to be released into the Fallopian tube. The ovulated egg enters the Fallopian tube and travels towards the uterus. It is during this journey that the egg may be fertilized. If not, some 14 days after ovulation the lining of the uterus is shed into the vagina – that is, the woman has her period. Then the entire cycle begins again.

CONCEPTION AND HORMONES

Hormones are chemicals that the body produces to regulate all kinds of natural processes. They act as messengers, telling the ovaries, for example, when to release an egg.

Two hormones play a crucial role in ovulation and pregnancy. Each month, follicle-stimulating hormone (FSH) stimulates an egg to mature, then luteinizing hormone (LH) causes the egg to be released into the Fallopian tubes, where it is ready to be fertilized. The hormones FSH and LH are produced in the brain, in an organ called the pituitary gland. The cells around the egg produce two other hormones – oestrogen and progesterone. These hormones cause the lining of the uterus to thicken, to create an environment in which an implanted, fertilized egg can thrive and grow. It is the monthly drop in the level of progesterone which, in the absence of a fertilized egg, brings on a woman's period.

The regular ebb and flow of different hormones throughout the menstrual cycle means that there are only a few days in each month when a woman is likely to conceive. This 'window of opportunity' is known as the fertile period.

FEMALE REPRODUCTIVE SYSTEM

The woman's egg is released from the ovary. It travels down the Fallopian tube to the uterus.

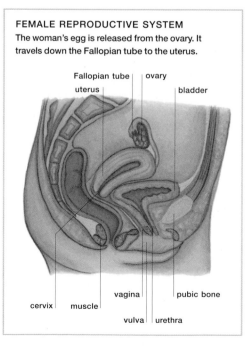

Fallopian tube | ovary
uterus | bladder
vagina | pubic bone
cervix | muscle
vulva | urethra

If the woman is menstruating but is not producing eggs for some reason, conception cannot occur. However, women can conceive even if they are not having periods – although conception is less likely.

THE MAN'S REPRODUCTIVE SYSTEM

A man's reproductive system consists of the penis, the testicles, and the various tubes that connect the two and carry sperm. Sperm is produced in the two testicles, which are contained within the scrotum. Men do not start making sperm until they reach puberty.

Thousands of microscopic tubes within the testicles connect to the two tubes, which are known as the efferent ducts. These lead into one single tube, the epididymis. The epididymis is part of the route through which sperm leaves the man's body. It is about 12 metres (40 feet) in length, and is narrower than a fine piece of thread.

THE SPERM'S JOURNEY

Men, unlike women, are physiologically primed to reproduce at any time, and so sperm are in constant production. A series of muscular contractions in the wall of the epididymis serves to transport them along its length. During this time, the sperm are modified so that they become capable of fertilization. They also acquire their ability to move (which is known medically as motility) while they are in the epididymis. The sperm now pass

> " Seven days after fertilization, the egg becomes implanted in the lining of the uterus. This is the moment when conception is said to take place. "

through a tube called the vas deferens, which moves them quickly into the urethra, which passes through the penis. The urethra is the tube through which urine is passed out of the body. During sexual arousal and ejaculation, the opening between the urethra and the bladder shuts, and sperm-containing semen is rapidly transported along it.

THE RACE TO THE EGG

It takes only one sperm to fertilize an egg. When a man ejaculates during sexual intercourse, between 100 million and 300 million sperm are discharged into the woman's vagina – at about 45km (28 miles) per hour.

Each sperm is genetically unique, meaning that no two contain exactly the same set of genes. The millions of individual sperm are now in competition with each other as they race to fertilize the egg.

The route to the egg is hazardous. This is why sperm are produced in such large numbers. To stand a chance of fertilizing the egg, the sperm have to be able to withstand the environment of the woman's vagina and cervix. The acidity of this environment protects against bacteria and potentially dangerous infections, but it is also inhospitable to sperm. Weak or damaged ones will not make it.

In addition, the force of gravity means that millions of sperm simply leak out of the woman's vagina – as few as 5 per cent of them reach the cervix. Of these, only 200 or so make it as far as the woman's Fallopian tubes. Any sperm that make it this far have covered a huge distance that is, in terms of its own length, equivalent to several hundred miles.

The last few superfit sperm now proceed to the outside of the egg. Of these sperm, just one will break through the surface, leaving its tail behind. This is the moment of fertilization. In the instant that it occurs, the egg's surface becomes impenetrable to other sperm.

Fertilization of the egg may take up to 24 hours. It then undergoes a series of complex changes until eventually, seven days after fertilization, it becomes implanted in the lining of the uterus. This is the moment when conception is said to take place.

Sperm can survive for quite a long time inside the woman's body – perhaps up to 48 hours – so fertilization can still take place even if the egg is not ready when they first reach the Fallopian tube.

MALE REPRODUCTIVE SYSTEM
Sperm travels from the testicles through the epididymis, vas deferens and urethra to the penis.

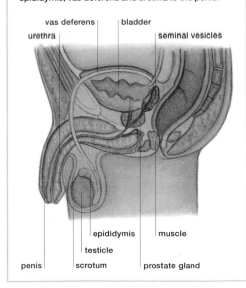

vas deferens | bladder
urethra | seminal vesicles

epididymis | muscle
testicle
penis | scrotum | prostate gland

Aiding conception

A baby can be conceived only around the time of ovulation, during the woman's fertile period. The egg is usually fertilized by the man's sperm within 48 hours of being released by the ovary. There are various ways in which a woman can judge when she is ovulating. By identifying this fertile period a couple can make a point of having intercourse and maximize the chance of conceiving.

WHEN DO I OVULATE?
Women ovulate about 14 days before the start of their next period. This is not the same as saying that ovulation takes place 14 days after the last period because the length of the menstrual cycle varies. Women may have a cycle as short as 21 days or as long as 38 days rather than the standard 28-day cycle.

There are various methods that you can use to calculate when ovulation is likely to occur. However, bear in mind that these serve as a rough guide only. Many experts and researchers in the field of infertility are sceptical about the effectiveness of the methods used. Even if you are certain that you know when you are ovulating, you should continue to make love at other times if you want to get pregnant.

Your menstrual cycle
If you have a regular monthly cycle, you will know when the next period is likely to start. Count back 14 days from that date – this is the day on which you are likely to ovulate.

YOUR CHANCES OF CONCEIVING
Conception is more likely to take place if:
- The woman is between the ages of 20 and 34; the ideal age is 20–25.
- The man produces healthy sperm.
- Intercourse takes place at the right time in the woman's menstrual cycle.
- Both partners are fit and well, and are following a healthy lifestyle.
- Both partners are a healthy weight, with a good waist-to-hip ratio (see page 49).
- Both partners avoid smoking, alcohol and caffeine.

Working out your probable fertile time means keeping a record of your periods for some months, in some cases up to a year, to establish the normal length of your cycle.

Cervical mucus
If your periods are irregular, you may be able to establish when you ovulate by studying your cervical mucus (produced by glands in the cervix's lining). Just before ovulation, it is transparent, thinner and more profuse, and takes on a jelly-like consistency, so that a drop will stretch between your fingers without breaking. After ovulation less, more milky coloured, mucus is produced.

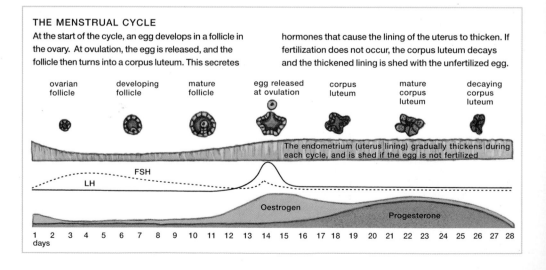

THE MENSTRUAL CYCLE
At the start of the cycle, an egg develops in a follicle in the ovary. At ovulation, the egg is released, and the follicle then turns into a corpus luteum. This secretes hormones that cause the lining of the uterus to thicken. If fertilization does not occur, the corpus luteum decays and the thickened lining is shed with the unfertilized egg.

ovarian follicle — developing follicle — mature follicle — egg released at ovulation — corpus luteum — mature corpus luteum — decaying corpus luteum

The endometrium (uterus lining) gradually thickens during each cycle, and is shed if the egg is not fertilized

FSH
LH
Oestrogen
Progesterone

1 2 3 4 5 6 7 8 9 10 11 12 13 14 15 16 17 18 19 20 21 22 23 24 25 26 27 28
days

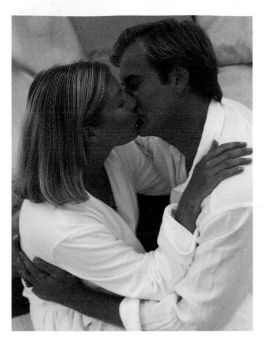

Making love around the time of ovulation will maximize your chances of becoming pregnant. All methods for establishing ovulation are approximate, however, so you should continue to make love at other times.

Body temperature

You can measure changes in your basal body temperature to determine when you are at your most fertile. Basal body temperature (BBT) is your temperature immediately on waking in the morning, before you have got up or eaten or drunk anything. BBT drops just before ovulation and then rises again some 12–24 hours later, once ovulation has occurred. If you record the changes in your BBT each day for several months on a special chart, a pattern is likely to emerge. You can use this to help you predict the time of ovulation.

Remember that your temperature can rise and fall for other reasons. For example, if you are ill or if you take your temperature later in the day, your reading is likely to be inaccurate. Doing both the temperature and cervical-mucus methods at the same time tends to give more accurate results than either method done alone.

Ovulation kits

You can also establish the day of ovulation by using an over-the-counter ovulation prediction device. These kits work by measuring the amount of the LH hormone being produced, which helps to establish when ovulation is about to occur. All you need to do is a urine test. If plenty of LH hormone is being produced, a chemical will change colour. This means you are likely to be ovulating. However, like all the methods, ovulation kits are not foolproof and can produce a false positive result. They are also expensive.

Remember that the consistency of cervical mucus may change for other reasons – for example, if you have an infection. For greater accuracy, it is best to combine this method with the body temperature method (see below).

To test your mucus, insert your finger into your vagina, then gently withdraw it. If the mucus is clear, moist and stretchy, you are probably close to ovulation. Making love within the next 24–36 hours could give a good chance of conception.

BODY TEMPERATURE CHART

In the temperature method, a basal thermometer is used to detect minute changes in a woman's body temperature during the ovulatory cycle; regular thermometers are not sensitive enough.

Most basal thermometers are supplied with a chart like this one. Make several copies so that you can keep a record of temperature changes over a few months. You may need help from an expert in order to interpret the results and pinpoint your fertile period.

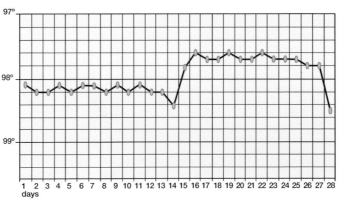

Preconceptual care

I deally, both you and your partner should start to prepare for conception a few months before you try for a baby. Nobody can guarantee you a healthy baby but if you and your partner are fit and healthy at the point of conception, you are giving your pregnancy the best start possible.

Your diet, weight and fitness can all impact on your fertility and on the pregnancy. Maintaining a regular fitness programme, eating a healthy diet and reducing stress can all aid your chances of conception, and will also help the woman's body to cope better with pregnancy. The months before conception are also a good time to give up smoking, reduce or give up alcohol, and attend to any other health issues.

The majority of women do not need any supplements other than folic acid either before conception or during their pregnancy. However, it is important that you start taking folic acid, which substantially reduces the risk of spina bifida, for a couple of months before you start trying for a baby – the current recommended dose is 400 micrograms every day.

DENTAL CHECK

Before conceiving, have a full dental check-up. Try to get any treatment done straight away so that you can avoid having X-rays or anaesthetics during pregnancy. Pregnant women are also advised not to have any amalgam (silver) fillings put in or removed during pregnancy since they may leak tiny doses of mercury, which is toxic.

MEDICAL CHECK-UP

Tell your doctor that you want to conceive. Ask about any supplements or medication you are taking – both over-the-counter and prescribed drugs could affect the health of your baby. Your doctor will also be able to provide advice on your diet, health and lifestyle, and advise you on losing or gaining weight, if necessary.

If you have diabetes, epilepsy or any other chronic condition that requires you to take long-term medication, your doctor may recommend changing the drugs or reducing the dosage before conception. He or she may also suggest genetic counselling if you or your partner have a family history of genetic disorders.

SEXUAL HEALTH CHECKS

Some sexually transmitted infections can affect your fertility as well as your general health. As they do not necessarily cause symptoms, you may be unaware that you have been infected. For this reason, all women

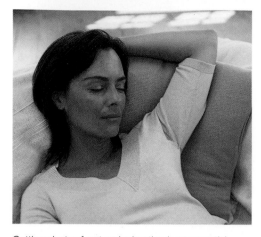

Getting plenty of rest and relaxation is an essential element of preconceptual health care. You should also make sure that you have all the vital health checks.

wanting to conceive are advised to have a 'well-woman' screening test. This checks for signs of:
- Bacterial infections such as chlamydia, gonorrhoea and syphilis, which can be cured with antibiotic treatment.
- Viral infections such as warts, herpes, hepatitis and HIV, which can usually be treated to improve symptoms.

Untreated chlamydia, in particular, is a major cause of female infertility and ectopic pregnancies. It may cause pain on intercourse but is often without other symptoms, so many women only visit their doctor when they have problems conceiving. Up to a third of people are thought to be infected with chlamydia at some point in their lives.

SEXUALLY TRANSMITTED INFECTIONS
Symptoms may include any of these:
- Pain in the lower abdomen.
- Pain during or after sex.
- Bleeding after sex.
- Spotting or bleeding between periods.
- The sudden onset of much heavier periods after starting a new sexual relationship.
- Pain when passing urine.
- Increased or foul-smelling vaginal discharge.
- Rash, spots, lumps, itching or ulcers around the genital area.

RUBELLA

Before you try to get pregnant, you should have a test to ensure that you are immune to rubella (German measles). Rubella is a viral disease that can cause severe abnormalities in babies if their mothers catch it during pregnancy. Have the test even if you are sure that you had rubella as a child – rubella is frequently misdiagnosed, and it is not clear how long immunity achieved in this way lasts. If you are not immune, you can be vaccinated and then retested to make sure that the vaccine has worked. You should not attempt to conceive for at least one month after the vaccination.

CUTTING DOWN ON ALCOHOL

Some doctors recommend that women give up alcohol before trying to conceive as well as during pregnancy, while others say that an occasional drink will do no harm. All experts agree that regular, heavy drinking or binge drinking can have an adverse effect on fertility and also carries high risks for the baby.

Up to two glasses of wine a week may do no harm during pregnancy, so this could be a good limit if you are trying to conceive. Spirits contain much more alcohol than wine or beer and should be avoided completely during conception and pregnancy.

Men should drink no more than two pints of beer or half a bottle of wine daily when trying to conceive. Heavy drinkers may produce weak, inferior sperm, which are unable to negotiate the journey to meet the woman's egg. They may also produce babies with serious defects.

Alcohol crosses the placenta, so a baby is exposed to alcohol when the mother drinks. An occasional drink may do no harm, but babies born to mothers who are heavy

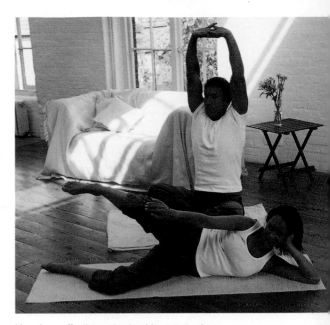

Yoga is an effective and enjoyable route to deep relaxation, and at the same time it increases your stamina, strength and suppleness.

drinkers may be affected by fetal alcohol syndrome. This can cause severe defects such as growth deficiency, facial abnormalities, problems with co-ordination and movement, and mental impairment. In addition, the babies may be born addicted to alcohol – and may suffer withdrawal symptoms and fail to thrive.

If you have had one child with a severe abnormality and are now trying for another baby, you and your partner should stop drinking for three months before attempting to conceive. You should continue to abstain from alcohol until you are sure that you are pregnant. The woman should continue to abstain throughout her pregnancy.

GIVE UP SMOKING

If you smoke, you should give up before trying to conceive. As well as affecting your general health, smoking reduces your fertility. If you smoke while pregnant, you have a higher risk of miscarriage and stillbirth; you also face an increased risk of having a premature or low-birthweight baby. Your partner should also give up to avoid the risk of passive smoking to both mother and baby. See your doctor if you want help with giving up smoking.

For optimum fertility and a healthy baby, it is best to give up alcohol entirely. At the very least, you should cut down to no more than two glasses of wine a week.

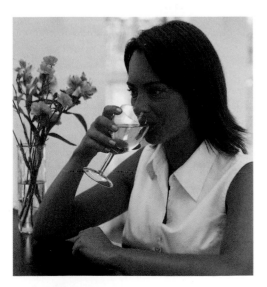

Time with your partner

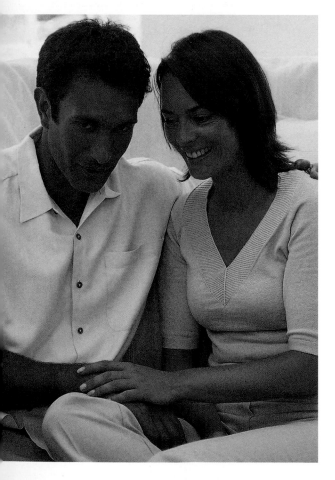

Before you welcome a new baby into your life, it is important to devote special time and energy to your relationship with your partner. The time before conception – as well as the months of pregnancy itself – can be a marvellous opportunity to strengthen the bonds between you, and to work through unresolved emotional issues.

It can be very easy for partners to become focused on the baby that they want, and to forget that they are life partners as well as potential parents. Couples who enjoy each other's company, and respect each other's strengths and aims, tend to make happy and committed parents.

A loving relationship and good communication can help you to face possible delays in conception as well as the challenges that pregnancy can bring. In the weeks and months to come, you may have to undergo a number of tests and checks. Some may raise difficult questions – for example, how you would react if there was something wrong with the baby. The time that you invested in each other before conception will help you cope together, as loving partners.

WORKING TOGETHER

The months before conception may be a good time to complete projects that you wish to carry out in the house or garden. Working together for the future can deepen the relationship and can also help you to prepare both practically and mentally for the likely changes to your lifestyle when you have a family.

Practical projects are also better done before the pregnancy is advanced, and certainly before you have a new baby to care for. Any unresolved long-term problems – such as clearing up financial affairs – would also best be dealt with now rather than later, when you will have less time and energy to devote to them.

ENJOY ONE ANOTHER

How you celebrate and enjoy your relationship with your partner will depend on what you both like doing. You may like to cook delicious food together, go for long walks in the fresh air, swim or exercise, have friends in for dinners and barbecues, or enjoy other shared interests.

Making love is, of course, a wonderful way to express your affection. For many couples, this is the first time that they are able to enjoy sex without having to worry about contraception, which can heighten the pleasure as well as the sense of connection between you.

SHARING MASSAGE

Gentle massage is a great way of deepening the closeness between you and your partner. It is also highly beneficial for pregnant women or those wishing to conceive. Anyone can give a pleasurable massage, and the basic techniques are not difficult to learn. You may like to enrol in a short course to learn from an expert. As well as being extremely relaxing, massage is helpful during pregnancy since it can alleviate common complaints such as backache, insomnia and even morning sickness.

Pregnancy can be an emotional time, with many ups and downs. A close and loving relationship will help you to face any difficulties together.

Giving a relaxing massage

The key to good massage is focus and feedback. Concentrate on what your hands are doing and enjoy the pleasure that you can give. Use the following basic techniques, alternating them in whichever way feels right to you. Ask your partner whether or not the touch feels good – or if they would prefer a lighter or firmer pressure. Then let your intuition guide you. Do not massage over a joint or the spine. Avoid using fast, rhythmic movements on a woman who is pregnant or trying to conceive.

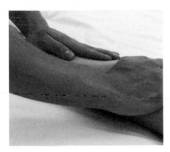 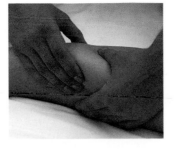 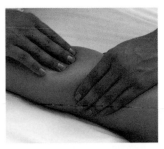

1 Start with slow, rhythmic, stroking movements, using the whole hand. Try applying light pressure with your fingertips, or use your thumbs or knuckles for deeper pressure. If you want to use oil, stroke it evenly over the area that you are massaging.

2 Gently grasp handfuls of flesh or muscle, particularly where you can feel that a muscle is hard or contracted. Use your thumbs and fingers to knead and roll the area, rather like dough. Keep checking that the touch feels good for your partner, and alternate with strokes.

3 Work specific areas by making a series of small circular movements with one or several fingers, the pads of the thumbs, or the heel of the hands. This helps to stimulate the circulation. Alternate with stroking movements, and remember to ask for feedback.

Aromatic massage

Adding a few drops of aromatherapy oil to your massage oil can heighten the pleasure and well-being that receiving a massage can bring. The main, immediate effect of aromatherapy is relaxation, which is very beneficial in conception and pregnancy – neroli or rosewood are excellent soothing oils. You can also use oils in a vaporizer, to create either an uplifting or soothing atmosphere in a room.

Aromatherapy oils can have a powerful effect and not all of them are suitable for women intending to conceive. See page 82 for advice on using aromatherapy oils safely and always seek professional guidance.

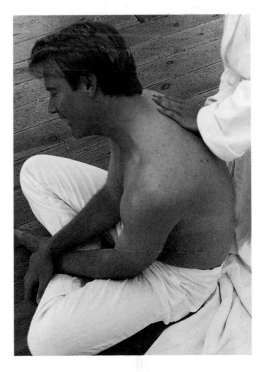

When not to massage

There are some circumstances in which you should not have a massage. For example:

• If you have an infection.
• If you have a high temperature.
• If you have severe back pain, especially if the pain shoots down the arms or legs.
• If you have a skin infection.

Massage is one of the easiest ways to de-stress and release the tensions of the day. It's also a great way to pamper your partner and enjoy time together.

Avoiding hazards

We know that some environmental substances, in particular toxins and radiation, may hinder conception and endanger pregnancy. The research currently available is not clear-cut, and it is by no means the case that all women exposed to a potential hazard will necessarily develop a problem. However, it seems sensible to reduce your exposure to hazards wherever you can, as a safeguard for yourself and your child. If you are trying to conceive, here are some of the things you should avoid.

X-RAYS

Having an X-ray exposes you to a tiny dose of radiation. The dose given is too small to cause problems to you, but it can sometimes have an adverse effect on the developing fetus. Always tell your doctor and your dentist if you are trying to conceive or know that you are pregnant. Wherever possible have any medical or dental investigations carried out before you attempt to conceive to avoid exposing the fetus to any risk.

If you had an X-ray before realizing that you were pregnant, talk to your doctor about the potential effects. In most cases, there is unlikely to be a problem.

OTHER SOURCES OF RADIATION

Computers, VDUs and televisions are sometimes cited as a hazard because they give out small amounts of radiation. However, the general advice is that the radiation you are exposed to in this way is not in sufficient quantity or strength to have an effect on fertility or pregnancy.

The research concerning the effect of mobile phones on the brain and the nervous system is not yet clear, but it would be wise to reduce your use to a minimum. Avoid chatting for long periods and use a hands-free model whenever possible. Do not chat with the mobile held next to your head while in an enclosed area such as a car.

CATS AND KITTENS

The faeces of kittens and young cats may carry the parasite toxoplasmosis. If this is passed to a pregnant woman, it can harm a developing fetus and cause a variety of abnormalities. The faeces is infectious only when kittens or young cats first acquire toxoplasmosis – which is usually while hunting during the first year of life. They then develop antibodies to the infection and excrete the parasite, in which case they are no longer infectious. To protect yourself, avoid contact with kittens and young cats wherever possible. Always wear gloves if you have to

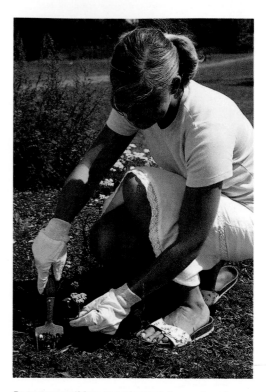

Protect yourself from toxoplasmosis by wearing gloves while gardening, and washing your hands afterwards. Check that your tetanus immunization is up to date.

TOXOPLASMOSIS

This is a form of infection that causes few symptoms – those affected may think they have a mild case of flu. So if you know that you have been exposed to kitten faeces, see your doctor for an immunity test straight away. This can detect antibodies to toxoplasmosis in the blood, and will help to establish whether or not you are immune. Unfortunately, the test can sometimes provide borderline results.

If toxoplasmosis is caught during pregnancy, it can cause a miscarriage. It may also cause damage to the unborn baby, including to the brain. If you have already been infected and are immune, toxoplasmosis will not affect future pregnancies.

> ❝ Complete any renovations before you try for a baby. Chemicals in some decorating products are harmful. ❞

empty a cat-litter tray, and disinfect it with boiling water for five minutes every day. There may also be toxoplasmosis in the soil so wear gloves for gardening. Wash your hands thoroughly after contact with soil.

APPLIANCES

It is worth getting appliances such as microwave ovens or gas heaters checked to make sure that they are working properly and are not leaking radiation or carbon monoxide into your home.

CHEMICAL PRODUCTS

Certain room deodorizers, furniture polish, oven cleaners, weedkillers and other products may contain poisonous substances. Always read labels carefully, and seek out household cleaning and garden products that are non-toxic and environment-friendly.

Take special care if you are exposed to chemicals at work – for example, if you are a hairdresser or a gardener. Talk to your doctor or midwife about whether or not any substances you come into contact with could be harmful to your pregnancy.

LIVESTOCK

Do not touch pregnant livestock if you are trying to conceive or may already be pregnant. They may carry bacteria that can cause miscarriage.

LONG-HAUL FLIGHTS

Sitting in one position for a long period – as you do when flying – increases your risk of deep vein thrombosis (DVT). In DVT a blood clot forms in the leg or pelvis. This clot can then become detached and travel to the lungs, a condition that can be life-threatening. It is now known that women are at greater risk of developing DVT when they are pregnant.

To help prevent DVT, get up from your seat every hour or so and move around. At regular intervals in between, flex your wrists and ankles and stretch your neck to left, to right and downwards in order to keep freshly oxygenated blood flowing around the body. Drink plenty of water before, during and after the flight – dehydration has been shown to increase the risk of DVT – and make sure that you do not drink any alcohol.

Home renovations are best done before you start trying for a baby. Choose products that are environment-friendly, to reduce your exposure to toxic substances.

IS YOUR HOME SAFE?

Take time before trying to conceive to make sure your home is a safe place to be. This is a good time to get done any jobs that could expose you to risk in pregnancy – for example, stripping old, lead-based paint from walls. Try to complete any renovations before you try for a baby – chemicals in some home-decorating products, such as paint thinners, strippers and glues are potentially harmful. Wherever possible, choose paints and other products that are child- and environment-friendly.

Many women find it difficult to bend down even early on in their pregnancies, so it is a good idea to complete any jobs that will require you to do so before conceiving. You should also fix any obvious hazards such as loose carpeting on the stairs.

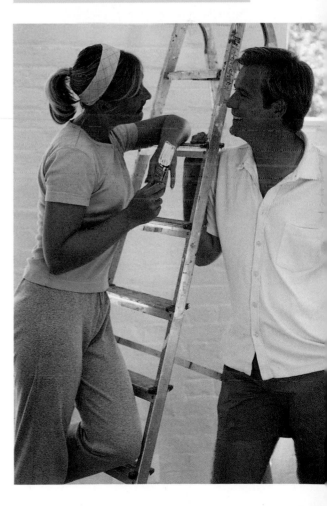

Common Qs and As

Q: How will having a baby change our lives?

A: Almost every aspect of your lifestyle will change to a greater or lesser extent when you have a child to look after. You will have to consider the child as well as yourself in every decision that you make, whether short or long term. For example, whenever you go out of the house, you will have to take a bag with extra clothing, spare nappies and other equipment with you. You may need to wait until the baby has fed, slept or been changed. You will be unable to go to some places, such as the cinema and theatre, with the baby – for those you will need to hire a babysitter or arrange for a friend or relative to look after the baby for you. In general, spontaneous outings will be much more difficult to achieve.

Although you will have less disposable cash and less free time, you will probably find that you will enjoy spending money on the baby and relish the time that you have with him or her. Parenthood often brings with it a very profound change in attitudes and priorities. You may find that your feelings about your career change and that you want to prioritize family life over your work. It may be that you start to feel that you have less in common with certain friends and that you actively seek out other parents to spend time with, or become closer to your family. Whatever the changes in store, many parents say that the joy of having a baby and bringing up a child profoundly outweighs the sacrifices they make.

Q: Once I have a baby, will I ever have time for myself again?

A: You will, but it will take more organization than before, and you will need the help of others to make sure you get it. It is a good idea to persuade your partner or a member of your family or a close friend to look after the baby for a few hours each week to make sure that you get your valuable 'me' time.

Q: My partner is very keen to have a baby and believes that it is a part of any normal human relationship to have children together. I am not so sure... and I don't know what to do.

A: You could say that it is part of most human partnerships to have a baby, but not all. There is nothing abnormal in not having children of your own. If you have doubts about having a child, give yourself and your partner more time to think things over. You may come to realize that your doubts simply reflect a certain anxiety on your part about how you will adapt to parenthood. You may also realize that there are other things you want to do with your life before you have children. Over time, you may discover that you are prepared to welcome this new challenge.

Q: My sister-in-law tells me that having children is nothing but drudgery. She says that if she had known what it is like, she would have thought twice about having her children at all. What do you think?

A: It may be that you caught your sister-in-law at a bad time. Perhaps she was feeling tired after work and knew she was behind with all the washing and housework. It may be that she thought back to her single life, before children, and wished for the luxury of time to herself. If you talked to her again, you might discover that she is happy and proud of her children and would not be without them. On the other hand, it may be that she really does yearn for the apparent freedom and luxury of a child-free life. It is important to remember that what someone else feels is no indication of how you would react in a similar situation.

Q : My mother and my mother-in-law keep telling us that it is best to have children as young as possible. We would like to wait for a few years. Is this safe?

A : The ideal time to conceive is in your twenties. However, many women are having babies in their early thirties without problems. It is only after the age of 35 that a woman's fertility decreases significantly. Should any problem present itself, it could take time to be resolved and, at over 35, time starts to be against you. That said, many women have healthy babies in their late thirties and even their forties.

You should remember that mothers and mothers-in-law are often eager for grandchildren, and this may colour their judgement as to what's best for their daughters and daughters-in-law. You must be your own judge; only when you and your partner feel the time is right should you go ahead.

Q : I am concerned that my partner is talking about giving up her job after she has our baby. I don't think this will be helpful for her sanity or for our finances. What can I say to her?

A : It may be that a compromise solution in which she works part-time is the best option for you both. You may find it helpful to sit down together and work out three different budgets: one based on her returning to work, one on her working part-time and the other on her staying at home.

Your partner will need to work out how much money she will need from you if she is to stay at home full-time. This will help her to appreciate the impact this has on your joint finances. Be sure to include everything in your budget, and allow for extras such as holidays. When you have completed the budget, add at least 10 per cent as a contingency figure.

Q : I have recently got married to a man who has been married before and has two children by his first wife. I do not have any children and would love to start a family. My husband is reluctant to have a baby on the grounds that it could upset his children. I feel that this goes against my nature and is unfair. How can I persuade him?

A : This is an extremely complex issue, made more tricky because it affects a number of people who are bound up together in a potentially sensitive situation. First, it must be said that if you really want to have a child but do not act on that desire, you could regret it for the rest of your life. So it is important that you make it absolutely clear to your husband how important having a child is to you.

Fathers who no longer live with their children, through divorce, often suffer considerable guilt and anxiety as a result. Once they become calm and settled within their new marriage, they are often much more likely to consider positively the idea of having another child. It will help if you tell him that you understand these issues and also that you are in no way trying to cancel out his former marriage by creating another family. Take positive steps to show him that there will always be time and space in your lives for his first two children.

Ask your husband if he would like to encourage some kind of open dialogue with his children, if they are old enough to appreciate the issues. You may also find it beneficial to have one or two counselling sessions, attended by both you and your husband.

CHAPTER TWO
Healthy eating

" What you eat will affect the growth and development of every part of your baby. "

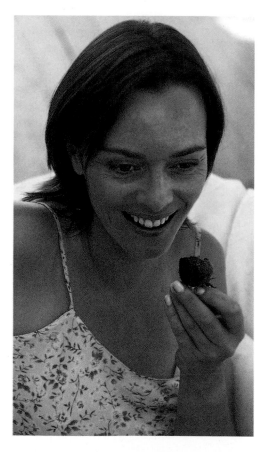

From the very first moment of conception, your baby will benefit from your healthy eating habits, as well as those of your partner. What you eat will affect the growth and development of every part of your baby: his or her bones, muscles, joints, teeth, senses and brain. Many people also believe that certain foods can even boost fertility.

Eating healthily and well is not nearly as complicated as some magazines and books lead us to believe. As you will see in the following chapter, good nutrition depends on a very simple formula indeed: eating a wide range of healthy foods and avoiding junk food.

Certain foods and toxins should be completely avoided before and during pregnancy and these are described in detail in the following pages. As far as supplements are concerned, there are very few – other than folic acid – that the woman who is pregnant or hoping to conceive needs to take.

If you get hungry between meals, try to snack on fruit rather than the many tempting – but usually unhealthy – alternatives that are all too readily available.

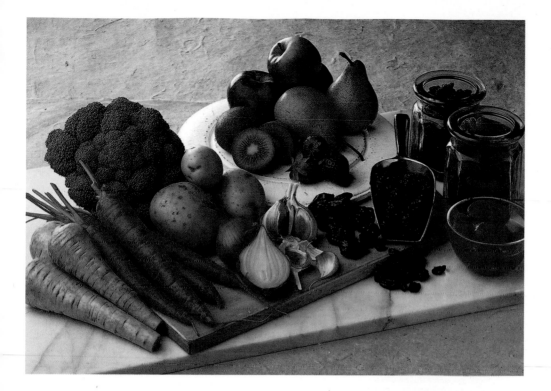

Food hygiene and how you prepare food is an important concept for pregnant women and is, in any case, something that all of us need to be fully aware of. Some food bugs may adversely affect the baby's healthy development and in some cases prove fatal to the unborn baby.

We have so much information available to us these days about the effects of food and how it is produced that all of us can take what we need for optimum health, growth and development and avoid harmful foods. Use this chapter as your guide to what and how much to eat and drink, what your weight should be, and how you can treat yourself to a cleansing detox day.

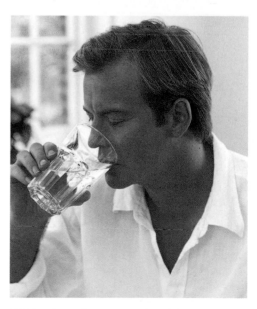

Top: A healthy diet is a well-balanced one, with a good proportion of fruit and vegetables. Make sure that you eat five portions of fruit and vegetables each day.

Drinking plenty of water cannot be over-emphasized. Even those of us who think we drink a great deal are probably not consuming enough.

Sensible eating

Healthy eating is a major cornerstone of preconceptual care. If you are trying for a baby, both partners should eat a healthy diet that provides a good supply of all the vital nutrients. This helps to boost your immune system, aids cell-repair and renewal, and keeps the reproductive organs in good working order.

Do not restrict your food intake in order to lose weight before conception (or during pregnancy). Dieting can adversely affect fertility because you may not be taking in enough nutrients to keep the body functioning properly and producing the necessary hormones. If you do want to lose weight, it is generally better to increase your physical activity rather than restricting the amount that you eat. At the same time, do not overeat. Being overweight and eating a poor diet have both been shown to have an adverse effect on fertility.

You should also ensure that you keep to healthy eating habits, which you can then go on to share with your children. Make time for meals, do not rush your food, and

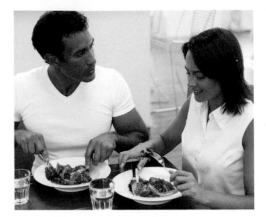

Make time to prepare and enjoy healthy meals made from fresh ingredients. Sitting at the dining table to eat will get you in the habit of taking good, regular meals.

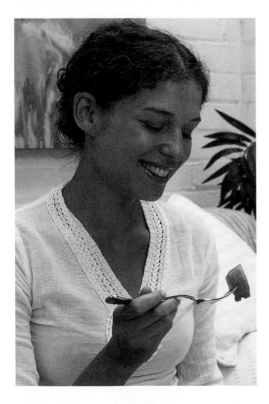

stop eating when you have had enough. Make sure that you do not miss meals. Eat little and often – having four or five small meals a day is much easier on the digestion than eating a couple of larger ones.

SENSIBLE EATING – THE WHOLE PICTURE

What you eat and drink just before conceiving will affect your baby's health to some extent and what you eat and drink during pregnancy is very important. Eating issues can't be neatly divided into 'pre-pregnancy' and 'pregnancy'. Mothers-to-be need to understand the complete picture of eating and weight patterns – both before and during pregnancy – to make proper sense of this vital topic, plus of course those women hoping to conceive might actually be in the early stages of pregnancy without knowing it.

Because of the positive effects of good eating habits on a baby's health, mothers-to-be were traditionally advised to 'eat for two'. Experts no longer regard this as sensible advice, but that is not to say that the opposite is true. Some women eat too little before and during pregnancy, in order to keep their weight down. Undereating can lead to problems such as more difficult labours and underweight babies and an insufficient supply of nutrients and energy to support the pregnancy.

Remember to eat at least five helpings of fresh fruit and vegetables every day.

ARE YOU A HEALTHY WEIGHT?

Here we provide two ways for you to check whether you are a healthy weight. One quick method is by using the chart on the right. Simply find the point where your height and weight meet and then check the key below. The other method (using the body mass index) is explained below.

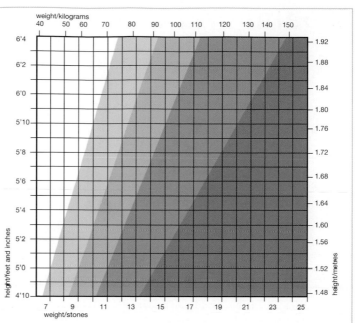

Key:

- Under-weight
- Healthy weight
- Over-weight
- Obese
- Very obese

Body Mass Index (BMI)

Healthcare professionals often use a calculation called the body mass index to work out whether a person is a healthy weight for his or her height. You can do this just as easily for yourself.

BMI = your weight in kilograms divided by (your height in metres) squared. (To convert weight from pounds to kilograms multiply by 0.4536; to convert height from feet to metres multiply by 0.3048.)

For example, Sue weighs 65 kg and is 1.64 metres tall, so her BMI is: $65 \div (1.64)^2 = 24.17$

A BMI of over 40 will adversely affect your fertility and is also a serious health risk. The ideal is a BMI of 20–25. Over 30 and you need to lose weight. If your BMI is under 20, concentrate on gaining weight through eating protein and carbohydrate, and having a full cooked breakfast and a generous lunch and dinner.

In general, women who gain a reasonable amount of weight tend to have easier pregnancies and labours, and a lower risk of miscarriage and neonatal death (death around the time of delivery). Heavier babies are often healthier than those with a low birthweight. However, pregnant women who gain an excessive amount are at greater risk of developing diabetes, as are their babies.

WHY WOMEN GAIN WEIGHT IN PREGNANCY

Women lay down fat during the early stages of pregnancy as preparation for milk production and breastfeeding. This fat remains after the baby is born, but should gradually disappear, providing you follow a healthy diet and exercise regularly. Other weight gain comes from the placenta, the fluids surrounding the baby and the baby itself, which accounts for more than half the total weight gain. During pregnancy, women produce more blood, and this also increases their overall weight. The extra blood is needed to support a healthy pregnancy.

Everyone is different and so there are no strict rules about how much weight pregnant women should put on. Most women tend to gain around 9–13.5kg (20–30lb) during pregnancy. However, someone who is already overweight may not need to put on as much weight during her pregnancy as a woman who is underweight. That said, the overweight woman should not try to diet once she knows that she is pregnant.

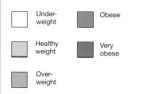

RATE OF WEIGHT GAIN

The following is a rough guide to the rate of weight gain through a normal pregnancy:

0–12 weeks	10 per cent
13–20 weeks	25 per cent
21–28 weeks	45 per cent
29–36 weeks	20 per cent
37–40 weeks	0 per cent

A balanced diet

Eating a balanced diet is a vital part of preconceptual care for men and women, helps women cope better with the demands of pregnancy, and gives a growing baby a healthier diet, too. Good general guidelines are:

- Include food from each of the main food groups every day.
- Eat five helpings of fruit and vegetables every day.
- Minimize your intake of animal fats and sugars.
- Drink at least eight glasses of water every day.
- Have regular meals.
- Choose natural unprocessed foods wherever possible.
- The only supplement that all women need to take is folic acid.

GROUP 1: BREADS AND OTHER CEREALS

These foods are excellent sources of carbohydrate, which gives us energy, and fibre, which helps to keep the digestive tract healthy. They also provide us with B vitamins, some calcium and iron. Eat whole grains wherever possible – for example, wholewheat breakfast cereals without added sugar, wholemeal bread and wholewheat pasta. Choose brown or wild rice, which have undergone less processing than white varieties.

GROUP 2: FRUIT AND VEGETABLES

Eat five helpings of fruit and vegetables each day. A helping can be a glass of juice, a piece of fruit such as an apple or banana, a small salad or a portion of vegetables. Fruits and vegetables contain a wide range of vitamins and minerals, have almost no fat and are a good source of fibre. Eat them raw or lightly cooked to gain their full nutrient value.

GROUP 3: MEAT, FISH AND ALTERNATIVES

Beef, lamb, pork and bacon are good sources of protein, which the body needs for vital functions such as cell-repair. They also provide minerals such as iron and zinc, and B

vitamins. Opt for lean cuts and trim off visible fat. Grill, roast or microwave meat, so that some of the fat drains off. Add more vegetables than meat to stews and casseroles to gives you a healthier dietary balance.

Fish and poultry also provide protein. Oily fish such as mackerel, salmon and sardines are rich in nutritious fish oils, so try to eat two portions a week. However, avoid eating more than one fresh tuna steak or two medium-sized cans of tuna a week, due to the mercury content (excess mercury can harm a fetus' nervous system). Grill, steam, microwave or bake fish rather than deep-frying it.

Nuts, peas, lentils, soya and pulses also contain protein but, unlike meat or fish, they do not contain all the essential amino acids needed for growth. To maximize their nutritional value, serve them with plant foods and whole grains such as wholemeal bread. Some people class pulses as a distinct food group, but nutritionally speaking, they cannot be considered as good for you as meat or fish.

GROUP 4: MILK AND OTHER DAIRY PRODUCTS

Dairy produce such as eggs, cheese, milk and milk products provide calcium, which builds teeth and bones, and some protein. Pregnant women need lots of calcium to build their baby's skeleton. Low-fat dairy products are generally better for you. If you worry about weight gain, reduce your butter intake and avoid cream. Natural yogurt is a healthy option. Women who wish to conceive or who are pregnant should avoid raw or lightly cooked eggs and soft cheeses such Brie and Camembert, because of the risk of food poisoning.

GROUP 5: FAT AND SUGAR

We need some fat in our diet. There are two main types of fat: saturated, which is solid at room temperature, and unsaturated, most of which remain liquid. Saturated fats, such as butter and lard, can increase blood cholesterol and

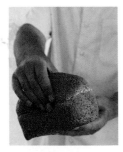

Try this test to check how healthy a brown loaf is: take the bread between your hands and squeeze gently. If it gives easily, it probably doesn't provide much fibre. As a general rule, the denser the bread, the more fibre it contains – so the healthier it is for you.

ORGANIC FOOD

Many people believe that organic produce tastes better and is more nutritious for you than conventionally grown food. Buying organic means that you are reducing your exposure to chemicals in the foods that you eat: organic fruit and vegetables are produced without the use of chemical fertilizers and pesticides, while animals used for organic meat are not given routine antibiotics or growth hormones.

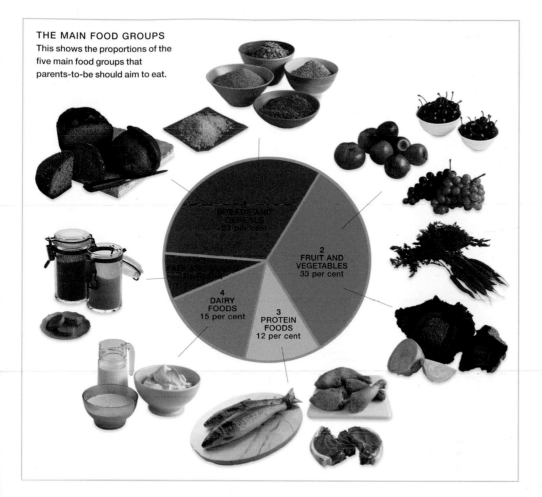

THE MAIN FOOD GROUPS
This shows the proportions of the five main food groups that parents-to-be should aim to eat.

1
BREADS AND
CEREALS
33 per cent

2
FRUIT AND
VEGETABLES
33 per cent

FATS AND SUGARS

4
DAIRY
FOODS
15 per cent

3
PROTEIN
FOODS
12 per cent

with it the risk of heart disease. The two forms of unsaturated fat – monounsaturated and polyunsaturated – are better for you and may decrease cholesterol levels. Monounsaturated fats include olive oil and avocado, while polyunsaturated fats include most vegetable oils, fish oil and nuts. As a general rule, pick low-fat dairy products and use olive oil in place of butter.

Sugary foods provide a short-term energy boost, but little nutritional value. Eat sparingly, if at all.

WHY WE NEED FIBRE

Fibre is an indigestible substance that we get from nuts, cereals, fruit and vegetables. It is not broken down or digested in the body, but is vital for speeding up the passage of waste products through the bowel and for removing toxins. Constipation is common during pregnancy, when bowel movements slow down, but plenty of fibre-rich food and water will help to prevent this.

DRINK WATER

Make sure that you are drinking enough water to maintain and repair all the body's systems, including the reproductive system. To avoid dehydration, which can lead to irritability, headache, tension, swollen ankles and a bloated stomach, you need to drink at least eight glasses of water every day – more if you are also drinking tea and coffee. This may seem like a lot, but after a few days your body will become accustomed to it.

Can foods boost fertility?

Whether or not certain foods can boost fertility is a matter of great debate. Some natural health practitioners strongly believe that they can. However, many doctors and other health experts profoundly disagree. Leading fertility specialists maintain that no food in the world can actually make you more likely to conceive.

To a certain extent, this is a matter of interpretation. If your diet lacks certain important nutrients, this could lead to fertility problems. A deficiency of zinc, for example, has been linked to low sperm counts. In such cases, eating zinc-rich food – such as eggs and whole grains – may help to improve the man's fertility. In general, however, most health professionals agree that following a healthy balanced diet, drawing on all the main food groups every day, is the best route to optimum fertility for both partners. Remember, too, that this must be combined with regular, sustained exercise.

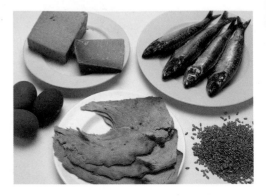

Foods that are rich in zinc, which is important for male fertility, include sardines, turkey, eggs, brown rice and cheeses such as Parmesan and Cheddar.

FERTILITY FOODS FOR MEN

Prospective fathers should eat a healthy, nutritionally balanced diet that includes foods rich in vitamins A, B, C and E, and essential fatty acids (which are found in oily fish and polyunsaturated fat). Men also need to eat foods that contain the minerals zinc and selenium.

Zinc and vitamin C play particularly important roles in the question of male fertility. Zinc is needed for the production of sperm and the male hormones: several prominent research studies have found that the male sex glands and sperm contain high concentrations of zinc.

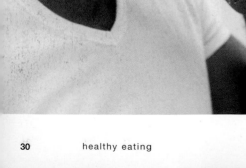

> **HERBAL TEAS FOR FERTILITY**
> Herbalists recommend the following teas, singly or in combination, three times daily:
> • cinnamon
> • cramp bark
> • ginger
> • ginseng
> • lemon balm
> • lady's mantle
> • motherwort
> • vervain
> • winter cherry

Men can play their part by sticking to five portions of fruit and vegetables a day. A glass of orange juice counts as one portion.

> " Drawing on all the main food groups every day is the best route to optimum fertility. "

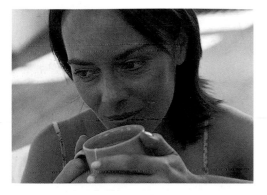

To enhance your preconceptual health, make sure you drink enough – but of the right kinds of drinks such as fruit juices, smoothies, herbal teas and lots of water.

Vitamin C is thought to reduce the tendency of sperm to clump together in the woman's body – a common cause of infertility. Modern diets are often low in zinc, and stress, smoking, pollution and alcohol deplete the body's levels further. Zinc-rich foods include oysters and shrimps, as well as other shellfish, sardines, turkey, duck and lean meats. Parmesan and Cheddar cheese are good sources of zinc, as are eggs, wholegrains, brown rice and nuts.

Citrus fruits, strawberries, kiwi fruit and peppers are excellent sources of vitamin C and should be included as part of your five servings of fruit and vegetables a day. Citrus fruits also provide selenium, another nutrient needed for fertility. One of the best sources of vitamin A is liver (not to be eaten by pregnant women or those trying to conceive); it is also found in egg yolks, dairy products, carrots, red peppers and leafy vegetables. You can get B vitamins from meat, green vegetables and wholegrains. Vitamin E is found in nuts and most vegetable oils.

FERTILITY FOODS FOR WOMEN

Any woman who is wanting to conceive should ensure that she follows a balanced, healthy diet. This diet should include foods rich in fatty acids, vitamin C, zinc, iron and folic acid – all easy to obtain from everyday foods. Iron-rich foods include meat, fish, eggs, dark green leafy

The best way to up your intake of vitamin C is to eat as much fruit as possible. Take melon, for example, for breakfast with muesli or as an after-dinner dessert.

vegetables and dried fruit. Good supplies of folic acid are found in green leafy vegetables, and also in nuts and pulses (see also pages 32–3).

If you have been taking the contraceptive pill, it may be helpful to increase your intake of foods containing the mineral manganese (good sources include oats, rye bread and peas) and also vitamin B6 (green vegetables and wholegrain cereals). These foods help to break down oestrogen, an excess of which may be associated with infertility. Eating zinc-rich foods might also be helpful (although shellfish should be avoided).

KEEP IT FRESH AND RAW

Another vital aspect of healthy eating is choosing fresh, unprocessed foods. There is still much research to be done on the effects of an over-refined, chemical-laden diet on fertility and pregnancy, but fresh produce, with fruits and vegetables raw or lightly cooked, is as beneficial to the prospective parent as it is to all of us.

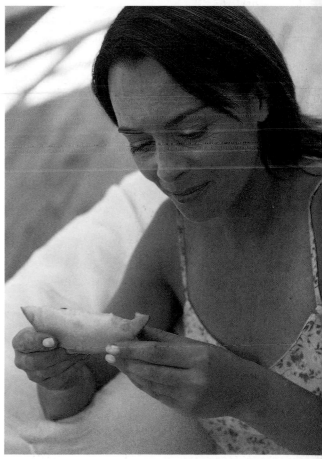

Do I need supplements?

You need more of certain nutrients before conception and during pregnancy. For example, your iron requirement almost doubles while your baby is growing. Many experts, though, believe that pregnant women and those trying for a baby can obtain all the minerals and vitamins they need from a healthy, balanced diet.

The only exception that applies to all women is folic acid. This is needed before conception and during early pregnancy in an amount that is difficult to derive from our food. You should not need to take other supplements, as long as you eat regular, healthy meals.

Some women may be advised to start taking supplements such as iron or calcium as the pregnancy progresses. However, this is only if they cannot obtain sufficient supplies from their diet; supplements are not needed as a matter of course.

FOLIC ACID

An essential B vitamin, folic acid (folate) cannot be produced by the body, so it must be obtained through diet or supplements. Women hoping to conceive and in the early stages of pregnancy need 400 micrograms (mcg) of folic acid every day, to help the baby's spine and brain to develop properly. To ensure that you are getting enough, take a 400mcg supplement daily before conception and for the first 12 weeks of pregnancy. You should also eat plenty of folate-rich foods such as Brussels sprouts, wholemeal bread and orange juice.

What folic acid does

Folic acid protects the neural tube – which will go on to form the spine and spinal cord – and helps it to close properly. This helps ensure normal brain and spinal cord development. Folic acid can help protect an unborn baby

FOLIC ACID AND THE NEURAL TUBE
Women hoping to conceive need 400mcg of folic acid a day, to ensure the healthy development of the baby's spine and spinal cord.

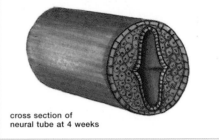

cross section of
neural tube at 4 weeks

from developing spina bifida (an abnormal development of the spinal cord) and anencephaly (absence of most of the brain). Infants born with anencephaly die shortly after birth, and babies with spina bifida are born with partial or total paralysis.

The neural tube should close between the 25th and 30th day after conception, when women may not realize they are pregnant. This is why all sexually active women of childbearing age should take folic acid each day.

THE ROLE OF MINERALS

It is important that you obtain a sufficient amount of all vitamins and minerals before and during pregnancy. However, some minerals have particularly important roles to play in the health of both mother and baby, so you should pay particular attention to ensuring that you are getting enough. Eating foods that are rich sources of these minerals is the most natural way of upping your intake, but some women may need to take supplements.

Calcium

You should make sure that you are getting enough calcium before you conceive because once you are pregnant the baby will deplete the reserves of calcium in your bones and teeth. Calcium is essential for the healthy development of your baby's teeth and bones, which begin to form from around weeks four to six.

Your body absorbs calcium more efficiently during pregnancy, and your baby is unlikely to go short. The baby will take what calcium it needs, but this may not leave you enough for your own requirements.

FOODS HIGH IN FOLIC ACID

• spinach and other leafy vegetables	• asparagus	• strawberries
	• Brussels sprouts	• bananas
	• orange juice	• grapefruit
• broccoli	• tomato juice	• wholemeal bread
• green peas	• oranges	

Folate levels decrease over time and with cooking, so do not store fruit or vegetables for long periods before eating. Cook vegetables lightly by steaming, microwaving or stir-frying.

CALCIUM-RICH FOODS

- milk
- yogurt
- cheese
- nuts
- sesame seeds
- pulses
- leafy green vegetables
- bread
- canned fish with bones (e.g. pilchards)

Make sure that you eat and drink plenty of calcium-rich foods before conceiving and throughout your pregnancy. You will need the equivalent of 600ml (1 pint) milk a day. A small pot of yogurt or 25g (1oz) hard cheese contain as much calcium as about 200ml (⅓ pint) milk.

Vegans and women who never drink milk, either because they are allergic to it or because they simply don't like it, may need calcium supplements. If you are eating well, 600 milligrams (mg) should be enough, but 1200mg may be advised in some cases.

Vitamin D helps the body to absorb vitamin C properly. This vitamin is found in milk, butter and eggs. More importantly, however, the body can manufacture its own vitamin D if it is exposed to the sun. You should therefore take a short walk outdoors each day to expose your face, hands and arms to daylight.

Iron

During pregnancy, your body manufactures extra blood, and your requirement for iron increases at the same time. You will probably need almost twice as much iron as you did before you became pregnant.

Iron is needed for the formation of haemoglobin, the oxygen-carrying pigment in red blood cells. If you don't have enough haemoglobin in your blood, insufficient oxygen may be transported to your organs and your baby. This will also result in your becoming very tired.

Make sure that you are eating plenty of iron-rich foods before conception, particularly red meat and dark poultry meat. Vitamin C helps the body to absorb iron from other, plant-based sources more efficiently, so it is a good idea to have a glass of orange juice or a tomato salad with meals. Another simple way of increasing iron intake is to use iron pans when cooking.

Pregnant women used to be given iron tablets as a matter of course. This should not be necessary so long as you eat a good diet with sufficient iron-rich foods (although

Take a short walk every day so that you receive exposure to sunlight. This enables the body to manufacture vitamin D, which in turn aids the absorption of vitamin C.

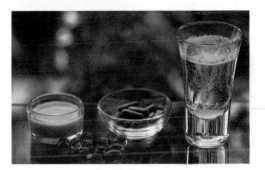

Supplements such as iron come in a number of different forms. Chelated supplements are said to be more rapidly absorbed by the body.

it may be necessary if you are expecting two or more babies). If you are worried about iron intake, or feel tired for no apparent reason, see a doctor. A simple blood test will determine if you are deficient (anaemic). It can be hard to get enough iron if you do not eat red meat, so vegetarians and vegans are often advised to take iron supplements.

Zinc

You need zinc to help the baby develop – there is evidence to suggest that an inadequate intake is linked to low birthweight. Make sure you are eating enough zinc-rich foods before conceiving; the body's levels of zinc can fall by as much as 30 per cent during pregnancy.

IRON-RICH FOODS

- red meat; dark poultry meat
- wholegrains
- egg yolks
- pulses
- nuts
- dark green and leafy vegetables
- dried fruit
- prunes
- dark molasses
- brewer's yeast

ZINC-RICH FOODS

- oily fish
- onions
- oysters
- meat
- eggs
- molasses
- pumpkin seeds
- walnuts and other nuts
- peas
- beans
- wheatgerm
- brewer's yeast

Foods to avoid and food safety

In the months before you conceive (both men and women), and during pregnancy, avoid taking in toxic substances if possible. You cannot combat environmental health hazards such as emissions from industrial sites, but you can make sure that you do not spend time in smoky atmospheres and that you avoid foods that may be harmful, are highly processed or lack nutritional value.

WHAT TO AVOID

The following substances may cause harm to you or your baby and should ideally be avoided completely.

- **Soft, blue-veined and unpasteurized cheese** such as Brie and goat's cheese, due to the risk of listeriosis.
- **Raw or lightly cooked eggs and poultry**, as hens may be infected by salmonella and other bacteria. Eggs and chicken must always be well cooked to prevent infection.
- **Raw beef** including steak tartare, rare beef and undercooked beefburgers, regardless of where the meat comes from, because of the risk of BSE.
- **Certain fish**, because they contain mercury, which can harm the developing nervous system in an unborn child. Avoid shark, swordfish and marlin and eat no more than one tuna steak or two medium cans of tuna each week.
- **Shellfish and raw fish**, which carry a higher-than-average risk of food poisoning.
- **Liver**, liver pâté and liver sausage. They are high in vitamin A, which can cause damage to the fetus.

OESTROGEN AND FERTILITY PROBLEMS

The female hormone oestrogen, used in some contraceptive pills, plays a vital role in reproduction. Research suggests that some women who take an oestrogen-containing pill for several years may suffer reduced fertility for a few weeks or months when they stop. Oestrogens are also found in non-organic dairy produce and meat, pesticides, fish from polluted waters, plastic containers and clear film (plastic wrap).

Increased exposure to synthetic oestrogens may be one reason for the rise in fertility problems. In men, too much oestrogen can lower sperm count, while an excess in women is thought to be associated with conditions such as endometriosis and ovarian cysts, both of which adversely affect fertility.

- **Unpasteurized milk**, which may harbour highly harmful bacteria, including salmonella and listeria (see also section on preventing food poisoning).

Minimize your intake of the following foods and drinks:

- **Alcohol**, which may impede the uptake of B-vitamins, zinc and iron, lower hormone levels, inhibit ovulation and the ability of sperm to move, and harm a fetus.
- **Tea and coffee**, whose caffeine content may harm female fertility. A lot of tea can impede iron uptake.
- **Sugary foods** such as cookies, cakes and other sweet snacks and drinks, which contain few nutrients.

BANISHING CAFFEINE

If you want to conceive, it is a good idea to cut out or cut down on caffeine, tea and chocolate. Researchers have found that they can have an adverse effect on female fertility.

One study found that taking in more than 300mg of caffeine a day lowered a woman's chance of conceiving by as much as 27 per cent. Even modest consumption appears to hinder conception: women who drink only one to two cups daily lowered their chances of conceiving by about 10 per cent.

Another study found that an intake of more than 300mg of caffeine a day may be associated with miscarriage. In addition, pregnant women who drank eight or more cups of coffee a day were found to have double the risk of stillbirth as women who did not drink coffee.

It is helpful if you have some way of measuring 300mg of caffeine. This 300mg limit is roughly equivalent to the following items:

- Four cups or three mugs of instant coffee.
- Three cups of brewed coffee.
- Six cups of tea.
- Eight cans of regular cola drinks.
- Four cans of energy drinks.
- Two 200g (7oz) bars of chocolate.

There are all kinds of non-caffeine hot drinks available today that form good alternatives to tea and coffee, from herbal tea to barley-based drinks.

- **Fried foods and junk food**, which are high in unhealthy fats and should be avoided where possible.
- **Salt**, from adding salt to food or eating salty snacks such as crisps (US potato chips). Excess salt increases the risk of high blood pressure, which can be harmful.
- **Convenience foods and takeaway meals**, as these have poor nutrient value. Eat fresh, natural foods.

PREVENTING FOOD POISONING

Poor food hygiene is responsible for thousands of cases of food poisoning every year. Most people suffer a bout of diarrhoea or sickness and have no long-term effects. However, women who may be, or are, pregnant must take great care to avoid food poisoning, as there is a real threat to the unborn baby.

Food poisoning is usually the result of eating food that has been contaminated by bacteria. These precautions will help prevent bacteria from spreading and multiplying:
- Wash your hands with hot water and an antibacterial soap before and after handling food, especially poultry, raw meat, fish, seafood, salads, vegetables and eggs.
- Wash your hands with hot water and antibacterial soap after handling cats, dogs and other domestic pets.
- Disinfect kitchen surfaces with an antibacterial solution, to kill potentially harmful bacteria.
- Use plastic, not wooden, chopping boards, and disinfect them after each use. Use separate boards for cooked and raw foods.
- Fridges should be kept at under 5°C (41°F). Use a fridge thermometer to be sure the temperature is right.
- Store raw foods separately from ready-to-eat and cooked foods (place raw meat and fish on the bottom shelf of the fridge). Always abide by use-by dates.
- Regularly clean taps, telephones and any gadgets in the kitchen, using an antibacterial solution.

Avoiding listeriosis

Listeriosis is caused by the bacterium *Listeria monocytogenes*. If caught during pregnancy, it can result in miscarriage, stillbirth or severe illness in the baby.

High levels of listeria have been found in some foods, so it is advisable to avoid these. They include:
- Unpasteurized milk.
- Pâté made from meat, fish or vegetables.
- Mould-ripened and blue-veined cheeses.
- Soft-whip ice cream from ice-cream machines.
- Pre-cooked poultry and cook-chill meals unless thoroughly reheated.
- Prepared salads, unless washed thoroughly.

Avoiding Campylobacter pylori

The bacterium *Campylobacter pylori* is the chief cause of food poisoning in both the UK and the USA – it accounts for more than 2.5 million cases of food poisoning in the USA every year. The bacterium is found in raw meat, poultry, wild birds and unpasteurized milk. This is one reason why pregnant women need to avoid raw and lightly cooked eggs and undercooked chicken.

Avoiding salmonella

Salmonella is a bacterium commonly found in hens. Be sure to cook poultry and eggs thoroughly when you are trying for a baby and during pregnancy. Do not eat foods containing raw egg, such as fresh mayonnaise.

Avoiding toxoplasmosis

Toxoplasmosis is an infection caused by a parasite that can cause miscarriage or damage to the unborn baby. It may be present in soil, so fresh fruit, vegetables and lettuce are all potential sources of infection. They should be thoroughly washed under running water.

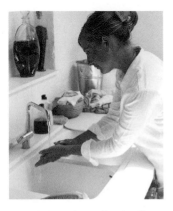

Be sure to wash your hands with antibacterial soap both before and after handling foods.

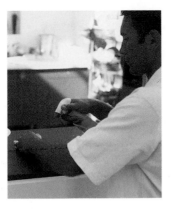

Always disinfect kitchen surfaces and chopping boards after preparing food on them.

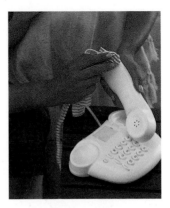

Use an antibacterial solution to wipe over taps, telephones and kitchen surfaces regularly.

A healthy day

You want to be as healthy and fit as possible before conceiving a baby. This cleansing programme offers a gentle way to eliminate toxins from the body without putting it under any stress. Undertaking a preconceptual detox with your partner can also be a pleasurable way to relax and spend some time together.

Some people associate detoxing with total fasting. However, it is very important that you do not take any extreme measures before conception and during pregnancy. Fasting is not good for the body, and should be avoided, in particular, by anyone wishing to conceive.

This programme emphasizes exercise, rest and relaxation together with healthy eating. Feel free to adapt it according to your individual needs. No special equipment is used, but you will need a soft-bristled brush for the skin, and essential oils of your choice.

A day of detoxing

Set aside a whole day – or even a weekend – for your detox. Choose a time when you know that you won't be interrupted, so you can focus totally on yourselves.

1 As soon as you wake up, drink a glass of hot water with a slice of lemon in it. Lemon possesses cleansing properties so will aid the detox process. (Drinking hot water with lemon when you wake up is a good habit to acquire.) Then eat a piece of fruit or a slice of wholemeal bread – don't add any butter or spread. This will get your digestive system moving.

2 Do some gentle stretching, yoga or warm-up exercises. Then, do 30 minutes of brisk exercise. This could take the form of running, fast walking or any other exercise that makes you slightly breathless (you should still be able to keep up a conversation). Brisk exercise speeds up your circulatory system, bringing oxygen and nutrients to all areas of the body and helping to eliminate toxins. Afterwards, drink a large of glass of water, and some juiced or liquidized fruit or vegetables.

3 Next, dry-brush your whole body in order to remove dead skin cells – either brush your own body or do this for your partner. Brush upwards, using long strokes on the arms and legs. Spend at least five minutes doing this, then take a warm shower. Use a body scrub to help slough off more dead skin cells in the water.

4 After the shower, deep-cleanse your face. Pour some boiling water into a large bowl, add a few drops of essential oil (chamomile, lavender or lemongrass are good choices), then place a towel over your head. Let the steam soak into your skin for a few moments, then remove the towel and pat your face dry. Splash your face with cold water a few times to tighten up the pores again.

5 You and your partner may like to give one another a massage at this point. Massage helps to boost the circulation, which speeds up the elimination process. Enjoy a full body massage, or concentrate on the legs and feet, where toxins tend to collect. A foot massage is easy to do if you are on your own and improving the circulation here will have a knock-on effect for the whole system.

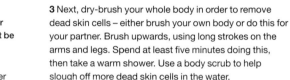

The most important aspect of detoxing is to drink water – and lots of it. Heighten the effect by adding a slice of lemon to each glass.

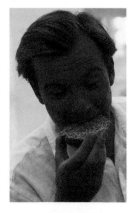

Wholemeal bread without butter is a wake-up call for the body's digestive system. Drink at least one glass of water, with lemon, beforehand.

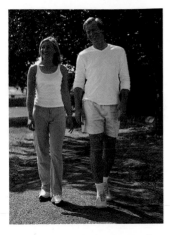

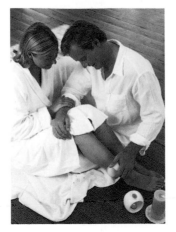

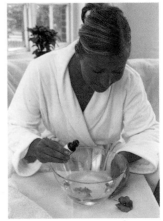

Exercise and fresh air are not only an essential part of detoxification, but are important elements of a healthy and enjoyable lifestyle.

Use a soft-bristled brush to energize your skin and remove dead cells. You and your partner can do this for each other if you like.

Give yourself a mini face treatment. Add a drop or two of essential oil to a bowl of boiling water, then allow the steam to cleanse your skin.

6 Spend some time relaxing after your massage; give yourself 30 minutes or an hour of total rest. Then do some gentle yoga or stretching to re-energize yourself. Stretching helps to mobilize the joints; it also increases the flow of blood, and brings nutrients and oxygen to different areas of the body.

7 Have a small lunch of fruit, vegetables and cereals. Stay sitting upright for at least 15 minutes after eating, to help your digestion. Then, go out for a short walk.

8 Do some meditation at this point, or simply sit quietly and focus on your breathing. Breathing deeply helps to get more oxygen to the muscles and organs. Wait two hours after eating, then do another session of exercise.

9 Have a salt rub. Waste products are excreted through the skin and massage, exfoliation and salt rubs all help keep the pores clean and healthy. You can use any type of salt mixed with a little olive oil. Rub into the skin with a circular motion, moving away from the heart. This aids the circulation and elimination systems.

10 Have a long aromatic bath, with your partner or by yourself. Dilute a couple of drops of aromatherapy oil in a carrier and add to the water. Afterwards, moisturize your skin. Combine this with another massage if you like.

11 Spend the rest of the evening quietly, perhaps incorporating some more yoga or stretching. Go to bed early to be sure that you get plenty of rest.

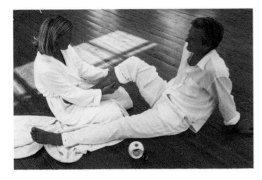

Take it in turns to give each other a relaxing massage. Try a leg and foot treatment, then a back massage.

ESSENTIAL ELEMENTS OF A HEALTHY DAY
Throughout the day:
- Drink only water. You should have at least 2 litres (3½ pints) and preferably more. Have a large bottle for each of you on hand so that you can keep topping up. This will also help you to monitor how much you have drunk.
- Eat lightly every two or three hours. Choose fibre-rich foods: fresh fruits, raw or lightly steamed vegetables, and whole-grain cereals.
- Remember that this is your time to relax – do not read, watch television or answer the telephone, and try not to talk about anything contentious.

Common Qs and As

Q: I have found all sorts of weird foods and food remedies for boosting fertility on the Internet. Do they work?

A: Most fertility specialists and gynaecologists would recommend that you eat a wide variety of healthy foods every day with plenty of vegetables and plenty of water. There is no need to single out any one particular food. Refer to pages 30–3 to ensure that you are not missing out on any nutrients.

Q: I have heard that detoxing is a necessary part of preconceptual care. Why?

A: Many people feel healthier, more active and invigorated after detoxing for a short period, say a weekend. One of the great strengths of detoxing is the focus upon drinking plenty of water and exercising, both of which are very good for us. However, a healthy lifestyle that you can maintain every day is likely to be much more helpful than the occasional short detox.

Q: I was anorexic when I was younger. Could this make a difference to my chances of conceiving now?

A: Provided that your periods have returned to a normal pattern, your previous anorexia shouldn't affect your chances of conceiving. However, in view of your medical history, you might be wise to consider a combined multivitamin and multimineral supplement. Check this with your family doctor, and make sure that any supplement you do take is suitable for pregnant women.

If your periods have not returned to normal, you should consult your family doctor without delay. If necessary, ask your doctor for a referral to a consultant gynaecologist.

Q: I have a very fast-paced job and tend to eat on the wing. Could this adversely affect my chances of conceiving?

A: Eating in this way may not affect your chances of getting pregnant, but it will certainly not help either. Eating snacks hurriedly is not a good or healthy dietary habit, and it makes it hard for you to ensure that you are getting all the nutrients you need. If you have any other underlying medical problem, poor nutrition will tend to exacerbate it.

You may like to consider starting to pace yourself now for life with a baby, by eating regularly and well. Snacking as you go will become increasingly difficult and impractical once you have a child to consider.

Remember, too, that stress can affect your fertility and your ability to cope with pregnancy, so you might want to consider slowing down your lifestyle as part of your preconceptual care.

Q: I don't usually want to eat much in the morning, as early-morning eating makes me feel a bit queasy. Now I am trying for a second baby, I want to make sure that I get into eating habits that give me enough nutrients. How can I try to achieve this?

A: First and foremost, ask yourself if there are any foods that seldom make you feel queasy in the morning. You do not have to eat standard 'breakfast' fare. If you find the only thing you can eat is chicken tandoori, so be it. Secondly, make sure you have plenty of fluids, especially water, and try drinking juices or smoothies, for their extra nutritional value. Thirdly, make sure that your other meals include plenty of protein foods such as meat and fish, as well as wholegrain bread and pasta, and fruits and vegetables. These foods will help to keep you going.

Q: I have noticed that most of my friends manage to control their weight gain quite well with their first baby. Once it comes to the second baby, though, some of them have blown up by three stone (nearly 20kg) or more. How can I stop this happening to me?

A: The best thing you can do is to exercise regularly for the duration of the pregnancy and afterwards as well – swimming two or three times a week is ideal. Mothers who are at home with the first baby may find it difficult to take time out to exercise. If this is the case with you, try walking for a good 30 minutes a day with your baby in a pushchair. Avoid high-calorie foods such as chocolate, biscuits, pastries, cakes, sugary foods, salty foods, fried foods, crisps, peanuts and alcohol.

Q: I shall be going abroad soon to a developing country for a long vacation. I am worried about what we eat and how it is prepared since we are trying for a baby. Are there any precautions I should take?

A: You should always take care with what you eat and follow good hygiene practices when travelling in a developing country. In particular:

- Do not eat snacks from street stalls.
- Do not eat any salads or peeled fruit or fruit salad.
- Do not eat shellfish, pâté, raw steak, undercooked poultry, raw or lightly cooked eggs, or soft blue-veined cheeses.
- Do not drink local water or have any ice in your drinks. All water should be bought bottled or thoroughly boiled before use.
- Clean your teeth with bottled water.

Check to see if there are any inoculations you need for your country of destination – and how far in advance you need to have them. Ask your doctor first how these could impinge upon pregnancy.

Q: There seems to be a new health scare almost every week about some food or other that pregnant women, or those trying to conceive, must not eat. I am becoming increasingly worried about my diet. How can I be sure that what I eat is safe?

A: This is a good question, but nobody can give you a cast-iron assurance that your diet is absolutely safe. The reason for this is that medical research, scientific research and research into nutrition is going on all the time. Scientists do make new discoveries, which they then publish. Newspapers can then seize upon this information and make the most of it – sometimes inflating it into scare stories. This can have the effect of making us think that none of the food we eat is really safe.

It is impossible to live without exposing yourself to any risk at all. The best you can do is to be pragmatic and to take precautions where you can. It has been well established, for example, that some foods are unsafe or carry a higher risk if you are or might be pregnant, so it is sensible to avoid them. These include raw eggs, liver, soft cheeses and some fish and meat. We also know that a diet including whole cereals, fresh fruit and vegetables, most fish, well-cooked chicken and other foods will give you a good range of nutrients, which helps your baby to develop. Making sure that you are following a balanced, healthy diet is therefore very important.

You should also take care to observe the rules of food hygiene. It can be a good idea to avoid eating out or getting takeaways unless you can be sure that good standards of hygiene are practised in the restaurant. Other than that, the best thing to do if you read any stories in the media that worry you is to have a talk with your midwife or doctor. They will help you to decide what, if any, changes to your diet you need to make.

CHAPTER THREE
Top fertility factors

66 There is seldom any need to worry if pregnancy doesn't happen right away. 99

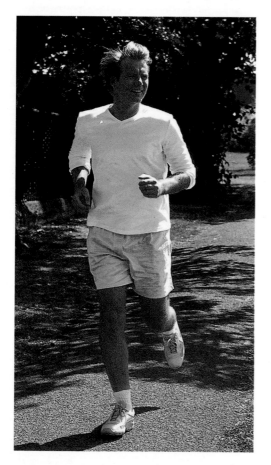

Some women become pregnant while barely thinking about it – it just happens. Others plan the pregnancy and find that they are pregnant within a few months. The remaining few may take well over a year to conceive and some of those may encounter a delay that is even longer than that.

There is seldom any need to worry if pregnancy does not happen straight away – this is very common, and many couples take the best part of a year to conceive. In fact, infertility is officially defined as over a year of regular, unprotected sexual intercourse without conception.

There are many ways in which you can boost your fertility level, as you will see throughout this chapter. De-stressing through complementary therapies is especially beneficial, both before conception and during pregnancy. In addition, you can prepare to eliminate the common causes of infertility before you even attempt to become pregnant. For example,

Keeping in good physical shape – and this includes your partner as well as yourself – is a key aspect of preparing the body properly for conception.

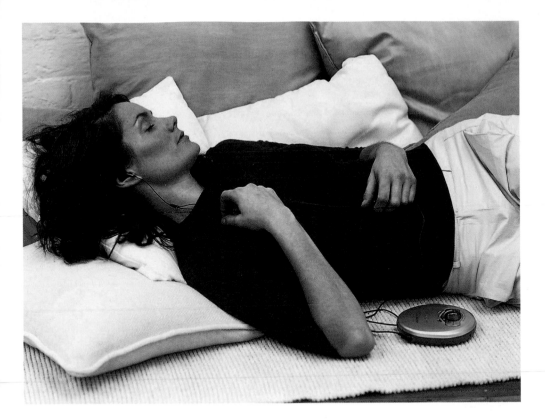

giving up smoking and cutting alcohol down to a very small intake are vital steps towards a healthy conception and pregnancy.

Your weight is another important consideration: extreme thinness and obesity adversely affect fertility levels in both women and men. As with everyone, attention to diet is the key issue here, combined with regular exercise.

There are also much rarer causes of infertility, such as inherited diseases. In these cases, specialist genetic counselling may provide the way forward, and is readily available.

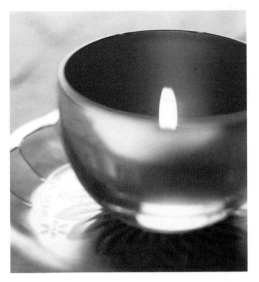

Top: Listening to soothing music is a really easy way to relax and unwind – it is thought that stress is a common cause of decreased fertility.

Simply using candles to create soft light and a calm atmosphere is another way to alleviate the build-up of stress that can creep up on all of us.

Getting pregnant

The best way of achieving a healthy pregnancy is to have sex as frequently as possible during the woman's fertile period, and for both partners to look at all the aspects of their lifestyle with a view to achieving optimum health and vitality.

HOW OFTEN SHOULD YOU HAVE SEX?
It used to be thought that a man would produce weaker sperm if he had sex very frequently. However, doctors now know that this is a myth, and so there is nothing to gain by you and your partner abstaining from sex with a view to producing more vigorous sperm. In fact, it is now well established that the more often you make love, the better the chance you have of getting pregnant.

Statistically, the chances of becoming pregnant in any one act of intercourse are low. However, you can increase your chances of conception by making love every day during the woman's fertile period. It is important to remember that many experts and researchers in the field of infertility are sceptical about the effectiveness of the various methods for calculating the fertile period. So, even if you think that you know when your fertile period is, you should still continue to have regular, unprotected sex at other times.

HOW LONG WILL IT TAKE TO CONCEIVE?
One important study into conception found that couples having sex once a month between the woman's periods took an average of 43 months in which to conceive. With couples having sex three times a month, the average time for conception was 15 months. If the couple made love ten times a month, the average delay was reduced

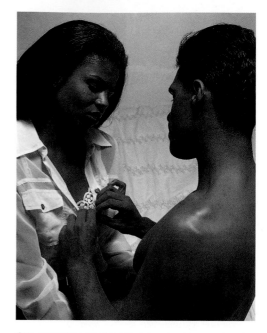

Give yourselves plenty of time to enjoy happy, relaxed lovemaking. The more often that you have sex, the more likely you are to conceive.

to five months. In couples who had sex 15 times or more each month, conception took an average of just three and a half months.

About one in six couples experience some delay or difficulty in becoming pregnant. You should not worry if it takes time for you to conceive, provided that the delay has not continued for more than a year. However, you should ensure that you are making love at least every other day during the woman's fertile period. Eighteen out of every twenty couples who are trying for a baby manage to achieve a pregnancy within a year. Another one in twenty conceives within two years. Others may succeed after trying for more than two years.

Nobody knows why conception can sometimes take a long time, or sometimes fail to happen at all. Many couples who have been trying for a year or two to become pregnant are perfectly healthy and have no obvious fertility problems. Ultimately, you may have to accept that conceiving a baby involves an element of chance – and it sometimes takes time.

THE PILL AND YOUR FERTILITY
Some women experience a delay in conception if they have been taking the Pill before they start trying for a baby. The majority of women find that their periods return to normal within three months of stopping the contraceptive pill, but a few may find it takes longer. If you are planning to conceive in the near future, some experts recommend that you stop the Pill and use alternative methods of contraception for three months before you try to get pregnant.

> **There is nothing to gain by abstaining from sex with a view to producing more vigorous sperm.**

EMOTIONAL FACTORS

It is often impossible to know why a woman does not conceive, but it is certain that emotional factors and stress as well as medical problems can play a part. Events such as moving house, starting a new job or suffering a bereavement in the family can all cause stress. This can reduce your desire to make love, and can also have a temporary effect on your fertility.

Sometimes the very fact that couples are trying for a baby can cause anxiety and so delay the wished-for conception. This is what lies behind the stories everyone has heard of couples who stop trying, and then quickly find that they conceive.

WHEN TO SEEK HELP

Medically, infertility is defined as the inability to conceive after more than a year of regular, unprotected sexual intercourse. You and your partner should see a doctor together if you have not conceived within a year of starting to try – or earlier if you think there may be a medical reason for the delayed conception.

It is a good idea to take a record of the start and finish dates of each period from the time that you started to attempt conception. This will help your GP and any specialist to understand your normal cycle.

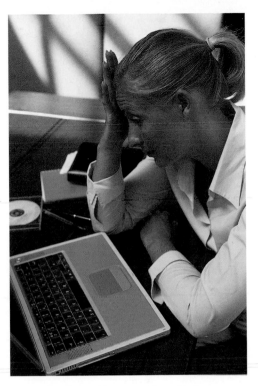

Feeling overwhelmed by your work can hinder your chances of conception – you may be too busy to make love at the right time, and stress can affect fertility.

Aside from medical problems, the causes for a delay in conception may include:

- Your age.
- Being overweight.
- Being underweight.
- Having a sexually transmitted disease.
- Drinking alcohol.
- Having a high caffeine intake.
- Smoking.
- Having intercourse at the wrong time – for example, being too busy to have sex during the fertile period.

Your doctor may give you individual advice on how to maximize your chance of conception, for example by helping to pinpoint the woman's fertile period or by advising you to, say, lose weight.

If appropriate, you may also be referred to a specialist for further investigations into the causes (see next chapter). Doctors do not usually refer couples for further treatment until after they have been trying to conceive for a year or more, unless there is a good medical reason to do so.

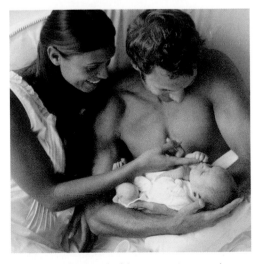

Eagerness to become joyful new parents can make delayed conception very distressing. However, many couples take more than a year to become pregnant.

Risk factors

Nobody knows why some women have difficulty conceiving, develop problems in pregnancy or give birth to babies with certain disorders or defects. But research has established a number of risk factors for pregnancy; these are listed opposite. Being affected by one or more of these risk factors does not mean that you cannot or should not become pregnant. However, it can mean that you may need closer monitoring and more detailed or frequent antenatal care than other women.

ASSESSING THE RISK

The many different risk factors may look daunting, so it is important to remember that over 97 per cent of pregnancies result in a healthy baby. If the medical staff involved in your care know of any risk factors, they can offer you appropriate tests and be fully prepared for any complications that may arise.

In some cases, women and their partners may benefit from genetic counselling before trying to conceive. Genetic counselling gives an individual assessment of your chances of having a baby affected by a congenital (developmental) disorder. This is usually offered to prospective parents who have a medical history that could affect a pregnancy. It may also be offered to women over 35 in order to evaluate the risk factor of age, and to women who have had three or more successive miscarriages.

HIGH BLOOD PRESSURE AND DIABETES

Established diabetes or high blood pressure can put the mother at a higher-than-average risk during pregnancy. These conditions can also develop during pregnancy, and this is one of the reasons that pregnant women need to attend regular antenatal checks before the birth.

High blood pressure

During pregnancy, high blood pressure is risky because it may lead to pre-eclampsia. This condition is one of the most common causes of miscarriage or stillbirth, so it needs to be carefully monitored by medical staff. Pre-eclampsia also poses a risk to the mother since it can lead to eclampsia, a serious condition that causes convulsions and can be fatal.

Symptoms include high blood pressure, swelling (in the face, ankles, wrists and sometimes all over the body) and the appearance of protein in the urine. This is one reason why urine is tested as part of a woman's antenatal care. Pre-eclampsia often develops at 30–34 weeks' pregnancy but it can start earlier or later.

Diabetes

There is no reason why women with diabetes should not bear a child, but they need careful supervision to ensure that their blood sugar and insulin levels are kept under control. Because of this, diabetic women are likely to attend antenatal clinics more frequently than usual. They usually have repeated blood and urine tests, so any problem can be promptly identified and treated.

Women with diabetes have a greater than average risk of such complications as stillbirth, pre-eclampsia, urinary infection and excessively large babies. For these reasons, pregnant women with diabetes are encouraged to attend hospital antenatal care and to have a hospital delivery so that specialist medical staff are on hand to assist.

Pregnancy diabetes is a form of the disease that occurs only in pregnancy and clears up soon after the birth. It carries the same risks as established diabetes.

RUBELLA AND RHESUS INCOMPATIBILITY

Both rubella and rhesus incompatibility can cause serious birth defects. These problems are more common than genetic and chromosomal disorders. However, you can be screened before conception so that both hazards can be avoided. Pregnant women are screened for rubella and rhesus incompatibility as part of their antenatal care.

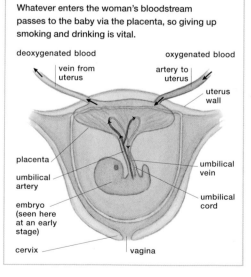

MOTHER AND BABY'S BLOOD SYSTEM

Whatever enters the woman's bloodstream passes to the baby via the placenta, so giving up smoking and drinking is vital.

deoxygenated blood

oxygenated blood

vein from uterus

artery to uterus

uterus wall

placenta

umbilical artery

umbilical vein

embryo (seen here at an early stage)

umbilical cord

cervix

vagina

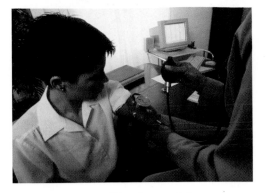

Your blood pressure will be taken regularly once you are pregnant, because high blood pressure can lead to problems in the pregnancy.

Rubella

Also known as German measles, rubella is a highly infectious viral disease. If a pregnant woman contracts rubella, the virus can attack the baby's nervous system and heart, causing deformities, miscarriage or stillbirth.

Rubella can exist in a very mild form and it is easy to mistake for a cold. Ideally, women should be checked for immunity to rubella before they attempt to become pregnant. If you are not immune, you can be vaccinated and then be checked again to make sure that the vaccine has worked. You should have the rubella immunity test, even if you think that you had rubella as a child. The disease is often misdiagnosed, and the duration of immunity acquired through illness is unknown.

Rhesus incompatibility

The rhesus factor is a substance found in blood: most people have it, and so are described as rhesus positive, but about one in six people does not have rhesus factor in their blood, and is rhesus negative.

Problems can arise when a rhesus-negative woman carries a rhesus-positive baby. In this case, some of the fetal blood cells can pass from the baby's body into yours. This provokes your body to make antibodies to fight the alien cells and destroy them. This reaction does not usually harm either you or the baby. The problem arises with a subsequent pregnancy if the baby is again rhesus positive. The woman's body now contains antibodies to fight and destroy rhesus-positive cells. These antibodies may pass into the circulation of the second baby and attack its blood cells, leading to severe anaemia, heart failure, jaundice or mental impairment. In an extreme case the baby would need a transfusion in the uterus, but women can be monitored for this situation and there are now injections available that help to prevent serious problems from arising.

FACTORS THAT MAY AFFECT YOUR PREGNANCY

The risk factors associated with conception and pregnancy include:

Age
- Being under 18.
- Being 36 or over.

Reproductive medical history
- Previous problem affecting the uterus, such as fibroids.
- Previous Caesarean or myomectomy (removal of fibroids from the uterus).
- Having an IUD in place at conception.
- Three or more miscarriages that occurred before existing pregnancy.
- Four or more previous deliveries.
- In a previous pregnancy, early labour, cervical stitch, late miscarriage, late termination, two or more terminations, stillbirth or neonatal death.
- Previous small or large baby.
- Congenital fetal abnormality in previous baby.
- Developing rhesus antibodies in previous pregnancy.
- Developing problems such as high blood pressure, proteinuria or pre-eclampsia in a previous pregnancy.
- Severe bleeding after giving birth to previous baby or manual removal of placenta.
- Very short labour (less than 2 hours) or long labour (over 12 hours) in previous pregnancy.
- Postnatal depression after birth of previous baby.

Other medical factors
- High blood pressure (140/90 or more, taken after you have been lying down for five minutes).
- Diabetes.
- Hepatitis B, HIV or AIDS.
- Family history of congenital fetal abnormality.
- Having a heart murmur.
- Pelvic or abdominal abnormalities.
- Being underweight or overweight.
- Being less than 1.5m (5ft) tall.

Lifestyle factors
- Smoking.
- Drinking more than ten units of alcohol a week.
- Illegal drugs taken by either parent.
- Having had a high number of sexual partners or a partner who is bisexual.

Race
- If you are of Afro-Caribbean origin, a test for sickle-cell anaemia is suggested.
- If you or your family is of Mediterranean or Asian origin, a test for thalassaemia is suggested.

What is the best age?

The best time biologically for a woman to have a child is when she is aged between 20 and 25. However, biological fertility is not the only thing that women have to consider when deciding when to try for a baby. Many women do not meet the person they wish to have children with until much later in life, or they may feel unable to cope with the demands of a new baby when they are younger. Women may also wish to concentrate on other aspects of life, such as building a career or ensuring they are financially stable, before they have a family.

Women's fertility decreases with age, particularly after they reach 35. Statistically speaking, both mother and baby also face increased risks as the years go by. However, it is important to remember that statistics give an indication only of the likelihood of a problem occurring in particular circumstances; they cannot predict what will happen to individual women. In other words, women over the age of 35 will not necessarily experience difficulty in conceiving a healthy pregnancy, nor are women guaranteed a problem-free pregnancy if they have children in their twenties. Many women have experienced the successful delivery of a healthy baby when in their late thirties and early forties.

AGE AND THE LIKELIHOOD OF A DOWN'S BABY The risk of a woman bearing a baby with Down's syndrome rises sharply as she ages.	
Age	**Risk factor**
20	1 in 2000
25	1 in 1205
30	1 in 885
35	1 in 365
37	1 in 225
39	1 in 140
40	1 in 109
42	1 in 70
45	1 in 32
49	1 in 12

PROBLEMS WITH CONCEPTION

Older women may take longer to conceive for several reasons. Most important is the fact that age can affect the general fertility of both partners. In addition, older couples may make love less frequently, and conception depends on regular and frequent sexual intercourse. At the same time, the menstrual cycle is more likely to become irregular as the woman ages, which may make it more difficult to pinpoint the fertile period.

One problem for women over 35 is that any delay or difficulty with conception may take time to resolve. If, for example, a 36-year-old woman tries to conceive, it will probably be a year before she realizes that there is a problem. She will therefore be 37 by the time that she seeks help. Fertility tests, too, can take time, so she may be 38 by the time a problem is identified. During all this time, the woman's fertility will have continued to decrease. Women who decide to undergo artificial insemination or assisted conception also discover that these procedures are time-consuming. In an ideal world, any fertility treatments and assisted conception should be embarked upon earlier rather than later in the woman's childbearing years.

AGE-RELATED PROBLEMS IN PREGNANCY

One of the most common concerns felt by older mothers is that the baby will have Down's syndrome, a genetic error that causes both physical and mental impairment. The impairment can be such that the child can never lead an independent life. As people with Down's syndrome may live to over the age of 50, this can place an exceptional burden upon the parents.

The possibility of having a Down's syndrome baby is not the only consideration for older mothers. Other risk factors that are linked to age include the increased possibility of:

- High blood pressure, which can lead to pre-eclampsia.
- Diabetes developing in pregnancy.
- Miscarriage and genetic defects – the likelihood of miscarriage rises with age in the same way as the incidence of Down's syndrome, but it is not known why this is so.
- Babies of low birthweight.

Women over the age of 35 are also more likely to develop other general medical ailments that may have an impact on a developing baby. Some disorders may need treating with medication that may be inappropriate during

66 Many women have experienced the safe and successful delivery of a healthy baby when in their late thirties and early forties. 99

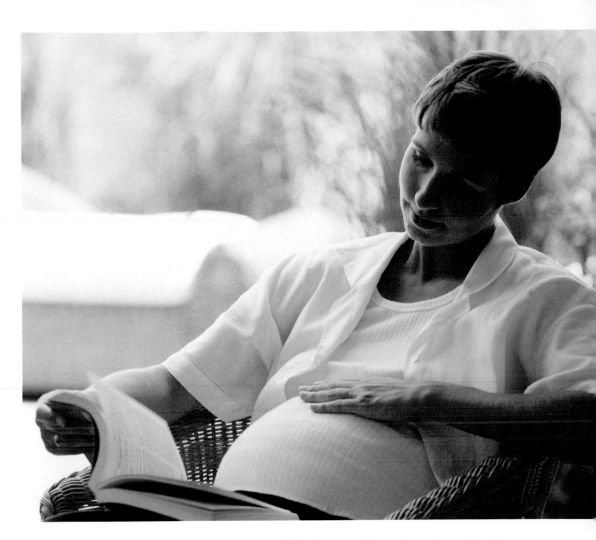

pregnancy. The mother-to-be may also feel very tired and suffer severe fatigue during labour. Pregnancy can also exacerbate any underlying medical condition, such as back pain or anaemia, because of the burden that it exerts upon the mother's body.

AN INDIVIDUAL PERSPECTIVE

All of this may seem highly alarming to the woman over 35 who is hoping to become pregnant. However, you should be aware that all the risks discussed here are based on statistics – your individual risk may actually be much lower. After all, a large number of women over 35 do have extremely successful and trouble-free pregnancies. In general, it may be that the older mother takes a little longer to conceive and that there are more potential health risks both to her and the baby, but the

While there are additional risks for older mothers-to-be, age brings with it an increased maturity and confidence that will be helpful during pregnancy and parenthood.

important thing to remember is that with good antenatal care risks can be identified promptly, monitored rigorously and treated.

When it comes to younger mothers-to-be, women under 20 may be physically healthy, but this is not usually the best time to have a baby. The woman's body may not be fully developed, she may not have completed her education and she and the father may not be emotionally mature enough to cope with the demands of bringing up a child. Young mothers also tend to be less aware of the risks of smoking and drinking in pregnancy, and they may be less likely to attend antenatal care.

Your weight

Research shows that women who are underweight or overweight may have difficulty conceiving, and there is also some evidence to show that men's weight can affect their fertility.

THE EFFECT OF BEING UNDERWEIGHT
Being excessively thin may be the result of restricting food intake or of exercising too much. Both can upset the hormonal balance in the body with the result that your fertility is affected. Women need a certain amount of body fat in order to produce the hormones that control ovulation. This is why women who are very thin may stop ovulating and having periods altogether. Men who are very thin may suffer reduced sperm count or function.

The best way to achieve a healthy weight if you are too thin is to add plenty of complex carbohydrates such as wholewheat pasta and bread to a healthy, balanced diet. Do not increase your intake of high-fat foods.

THE EFFECT OF BEING OVERWEIGHT
Excess weight in men can affect their ability to produce sperm, while overweight women may experience difficulty conceiving. Pregnant women who are overweight are at greater risk of suffering birth complications. Also, if you are overweight, it will probably take you longer to recover from the labour and delivery and you will be prone to fatigue both during pregnancy and during the first few months of motherhood.

All of the health risks associated with being overweight can have an adverse impact on conception, on the course

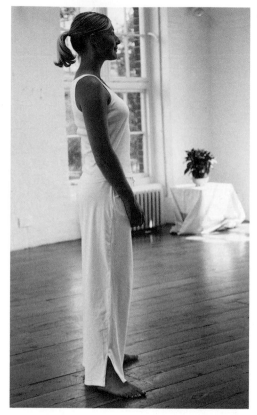

Being a healthy weight helps you to maintain good posture, which in turn reduces fatigue and aids the elimination of toxins from the body.

of the pregnancy and on the delivery itself – the most notable health risks in trying to become pregnant and maintaining a pregnancy are high blood pressure, diabetes and kidney disease.

LOOK TO THE FUTURE
Prospective parents may want to consider the long-term risks of being overweight, both for their own health and for the future well-being of their children. People who are overweight are more likely to die prematurely – and the risks rise with every extra stone that they carry.

If, for example, you weigh 85kg (about 13 stone) instead of the 65kg (10 stone) that would be ideal for your

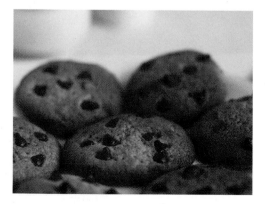

Being overweight reduces the chance of conceiving. If you weigh more than is ideal, cut out fatty, sugary foods.

height and build, your risk of dying within a given period increases by 60 per cent – statistically speaking, you are likely to die five years before your time.

All parents want to see their children through to a happy, independent adulthood. By looking after yourself, you will maximize the time you have with your children (and grandchildren) and the time they have with you.

CHECKING YOUR WEIGHT

The body mass index (BMI) provides a quick method of assessing whether you are a healthy weight for your height. Being under- or overweight may be harmful to your health and undermine your chances of conceiving. Check the box on page 27 to find out your BMI.

Your waist-to-hip ratio, which shows how much fat is stored in the abdomen, is another guide that you can use to assess your general health. To check your waist to hip ratio, divide your waist circumference by your hip circumference. The ratio should be less than 1 for men and less than 0.8 for women. For example, a man with a 80cm (32in) waist and 92cm (36in) hips would have a ratio of 0.88, which is fine. If his waist was 104cm (41in) and he had a hip measurement of 102cm (40in), the ratio would be 1.02, signifying he was overweight.

Both the BMI and the waist-to-hip ratio should be used as a rough guide only to your health and weight. If you are worried about your weight, it is a good idea to see your doctor for individual advice.

KEEP HEALTHY AND CONTROL YOUR WEIGHT

Diet and exercise should be the twin pillars of any weight-control programme that you may undertake. Natural therapies can help to strengthen and support your physical and emotional well-being, as well as aid weight control. If you want to lose weight, do so slowly and steadily – avoid any rapid weight-loss programmes, food supplements, diet pills or any diet that is based on a particular food group, such as all-protein meals. Ideally, you should reduce your weight to its optimum level and maintain it for several months before conception. You should not be dieting when you are trying to conceive or are pregnant.

- Eat healthily every day, and cut out sugar, salt, alcohol, cakes, biscuits, sweets, chocolate and peanuts. Your doctor may refer you to a dietician if you feel you need help with developing a healthy eating plan.

- Consider acupuncture to stimulate your energy levels, bolster your immune system and boost your lymphatic drainage system, which helps to eliminate toxins. A course of six or twelve sessions with a qualified acupuncturist may be the booster you need to set you on course for controlled weight loss.

- Try the Alexander technique, a system of posture and balance that improves energy levels, strengthens all the muscles of your body, increases suppleness and helps you to move properly. All these factors may assist your weight control.

- Use essential oils (aromatherapy) to enhance your energy levels. Some oils help to eliminate toxins and some help you to relax and thus improve your posture and movement. Always check that the ones that appeal to you are safe to use during conception and pregnancy before buying.

- Visit a chiropractor or osteopath, who can help to correct poor postural habits and so strengthen muscles. Manipulation of the skeletal and muscular system can also help to remove energy blocks – thus assisting the efficient functioning of the body's processes.

- Take regular exercise at least every other day, but don't exhaust yourself. Walking and swimming are good ways to start exercising. Dance therapy is a fun method you may like to try.

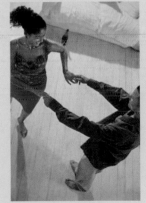

- Consult a herbalist for herbs that help to stimulate the lymphatic draining system and the elimination of toxins. Check that any you use are safe during conception and pregnancy.

- Try a massage or shiatsu. Both techniques can greatly improve the lymphatic drainage system. Toxins are eliminated and your vitality increases, which helps to speed up your metabolism and reduce hunger.

- Practise yoga for increased suppleness so that the muscles start to work at their optimum and your digestive system functions more efficiently.

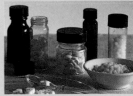

- Consider homeopathy, focusing on those remedies that help cleanse the system and relieve fatigue. Check that your choices are safe to use in pregnancy.

Fertility hazards

Smoking and drinking are two of the biggest risk factors for conception and pregnancy, but they are under your control. It is essential that you and your partner do not smoke at all if you are trying for a baby or if you are pregnant, and you should not drink more than a small amount before conception.

You should also try to avoid other harmful substances wherever possible. For example, avoid doing anything that brings you into contact with toxic substances and do not take any medication or supplements without discussing this with your doctor. In addition, you should be aware of any signs of poor health that you experience, and see your doctor promptly if you think that you are ill.

SMOKING AND INFERTILITY

It has been shown that smoking by either partner directly affects the chances of conceiving. Both partners should give up smoking some months (ideally at least four months) before attempting to conceive. This gives some time for your bodies to recover from the effects of smoking and also allows you to cope with any withdrawal symptoms that you may experience.

Smoking in the first few months of pregnancy is likely to have a more harmful effect on a baby's health than any other aspect of your lifestyle. Carbon monoxide and other poisonous chemicals will cross the placenta from your bloodstream directly into the baby's. This may affect development, and may make the baby more vulnerable to infection and disease.

Women who smoke during pregnancy are more likely to miscarry or to have a stillbirth. If they carry the baby to term, the baby is likely to be underweight (this is usually referred to as low birthweight) and he or she is more likely to suffer with infections of the respiratory tract, such as bronchitis and colds, in childhood. The child's ability to concentrate and learn may also be affected as may be his or her capacity for memory.

If you are already pregnant and still smoking, don't be tempted to think that it is too late to stop. It is not. You can minimize the damage to your baby by giving up now. Nicotine is a drug that, like many others, is addictive, and it is undeniably difficult to stop smoking. Your doctor or midwife will offer you advice on good ways to quit. While you are doing so, it may be helpful to remember two things. First, if you give it up now, you will never have to go through the withdrawal symptoms again. Second, you are now doing your best to make sure that you give birth to a healthy child.

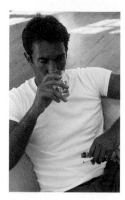

The occasional drink may do no harm, but both men and women should give up smoking before conception. Smokers and heavy drinkers may produce weak sperm that are unable to complete the journey to fertilize the woman's egg.

BREATHING IN TOXINS: WHAT SMOKING DOES
Tobacco smoke contains dozens of carcinogens. It also contains carbon monoxide, which is a poisonous gas that lowers the amount of oxygen carried around the body by the blood. Tobacco smoke also contains nicotine, which makes the heart beat faster and work harder than it should. Nicotine adversely affects blood-clotting factors, and so may play a part in heart attacks. In addition, tobacco smoke contains radioactive compounds, which are known to cause cancer. It contains hydrogen cyanide, which kills cilia, the tiny hairs that move together in waves to help keep the lungs clean and working efficiently. All of these toxins are entering your baby's bloodstream via the placenta each time you smoke.

DRINKING ALCOHOL
Fertility experts have different views on whether women trying to conceive should abstain completely from alcohol or merely cut down to a sensible level. The occasional glass of wine or beer is unlikely to cause harm, but most doctors advise women to keep drinking down at least to a minimum if they want to conceive. Two glasses of wine or beer a week is probably a good limit to observe, and spirits should be avoided completely. The man should drink a maximum of two pints of beer or half a bottle of wine a day, and preferably less than that.

If you are experiencing any difficulty in conceiving – that is, if you have been having regular, unprotected intercourse for a year or more but have not achieved a

*Strive for a healthy
lifestyle, good general
fitness and relaxation.
A happy, well-balanced
relationship is vitally
important if you are going
to create a new life.*

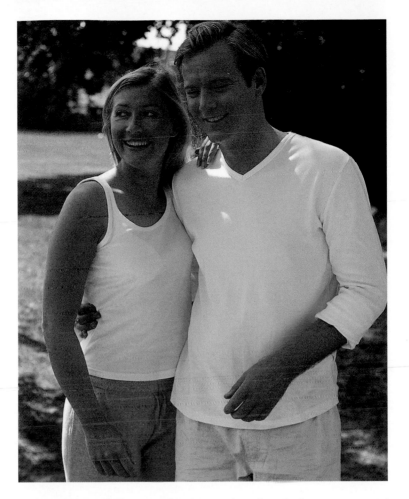

pregnancy – then both partners should consider abstaining from alcohol completely. Heavy drinking can affect both your chances of conception and the pregnancy itself. Men who are heavy drinkers may produce weak sperm and can also produce babies with serious defects. Women who drink excessively around the time of conception and during pregnancy can give birth to severely damaged babies. If you do drink heavily and wish to try for a baby, it is a good idea to see your doctor for advice. He or she may advise you to give up alcohol for several months before attempting to conceive.

YOUR GENERAL HEALTH

Ideally, both partners should be in good physical health before conceiving a child. This will give you the best chance of achieving a healthy pregnancy. A good level of health and fitness will also help the woman's body to cope with the demands of pregnancy and labour. It is

worth seeing your doctor for a check-up, so you can sort out any health problems before conception. This will also help to reduce your risk of having to take medication during pregnancy. Look at the list of symptoms below, and let your doctor know if any apply to you:

- Aches, pains and inflammations.
- Allergy.
- Apathy, feeling overtired, having less zest for life.
- Asthma or shortness of breath.
- Bloating.
- Constipation or other bowel problems, such as diarrhoea.
- Cough, persistent.
- Dark circles under eyes.
- Dental abscess.
- Fluid retention (swollen ankles, legs or fingers).
- Regular indigestion.
- Swelling and pain in the joints.

The role of the genes

Everyone resembles their parents. You only have to look at a family photo album to see how obviously and how often human characteristics are passed on from one generation to the next.

The mechanism by which these resemblances pass down the generations is the gene. Every human being has around 70,000 genes, and each gene contains a piece of information about one detail of a person's inherited make-up. For an embryo in the uterus, the data contained in the genes function as instructions: they tell the growing organism how to organize the multiplying cells into a human baby (as opposed to a frog or a rose); and they make that baby an individual, with a unique set of identifying characteristics inherited from its parents.

These genes are responsible for all that we are at the moment of our birth. They determine physical details such as our build, hair colour and facial features. Genes also govern, for good and ill, our natural propensities. A bookish nature, a gift for football, playing the violin or painting – all these talents can be learned, but they tend to be inborn. That is, somewhere in those 70,000 genes there is one for intelligence, athleticism, musicality or artistry that comes to a child as a birthday gift from its father or mother.

WHERE GENES ARE

There is a complete set of genes within every cell of a human body. Each drop of blood, every hair – every tear, even – contains millions of copies of the total blueprint for each individual. This is why blood tests can tell doctors so much about a person's genetic make-up: all the information about who you are is there to be decoded.

Genes are stored in long strings of DNA, and DNA forms part of the 46 pairs of chromosomes in the core of every cell. Every person inherits 23 chromosomes from their father (via the specialized sex cells in sperm) and 23 from their mother (via the sex cells in ova). The mix is random, and unique from the very moment of conception. Each child in a family gets a different set of 46, and so a different collection of genes. This is why brothers and sisters are not clones of each other.

WHAT CAN GO WRONG

Copies of chromosomes are laid down within sex cells, ready to be passed on to the next generation. But sometimes the copying process can go wrong and a gene mutates. This can have no effect at all, or it may result in an abnormality that manifests itself as a disease in the next generation. If that disease is not fatal, and the person

THE SPIRAL OF LIFE
Genes are stored in the double helix of DNA. There is a complete set of genes in every human cell.

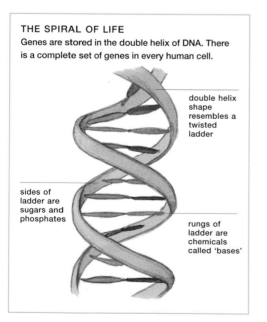

double helix shape resembles a twisted ladder

sides of ladder are sugars and phosphates

rungs of ladder are chemicals called 'bases'

INHERITED DISORDERS
Some of the most common inherited disorders include the following:

- Congenital heart defects.
- Diabetes, type 1.
- Cleft lip and palate.
- Colour blindness.
- Thalassaemia (blood disorder).
- Fragile-X syndrome (the leading cause of mental impairment).
- Sickle-cell anaemia.
- Cystic fibrosis.
- Muscular dystrophy.
- Haemophilia (blood-clotting disorder).
- Polycystic kidney disease.
- Haemochromatosis (iron storage disease).
- Achondroplasia (disorder of bone growth).
- Huntington's disease/Chorea (brain disorder).
- Albinism (lack of the pigment melanin).
- Marfan's syndrome (disorder affecting the heart, eyes and skeleton).
- Tay-Sachs disease (disorder affecting the brain).

affected grows up and has children, then the mutated gene can be passed on with all the others, perpetuating the illness in subsequent generations. So, a hereditary illness represents a tiny flaw in the genetic make-up of a person who may have lived generations ago. That person passed the flaw on by chance, in the natural way, and now it has become a fixture of the genetic make-up of some of his or her descendants.

However, there is another kind of disorder affecting the genetic process. Sometimes something goes wrong not with an individual gene, but with the entire chromosome. Some chromosomal disorders inevitably result in miscarriage, because some vital piece of genetic information has been lost. There are some chromosomal disorders which are not fatal or life-threatening, but do result in illness or some other medical disorder for the child. The best-known example is Down's syndrome, which results when an embryo inherits an extra chromosome from the parents, and so has 47 instead of the usual 46.

It is important to understand that chromosomal disorders are not hereditary. A hereditary disorder is one where all the genetic information has been passed on correctly to the embryo, but it just so happens that one of the characteristics that has been passed on is flawed or damaged from a health point of view. A chromosomal disorder, on the other hand, is one where the process has gone awry at the moment of conception. It is a genetic accident, not an inherited condition.

These disorders are rare: about one in every 100 births includes such a single gene disorder. Chromosomal abnormality occurs in about one in every 150 births.

WHAT IS GENETIC COUNSELLING?

Genetic counselling is a consultation with a doctor at which the possible effects of any genetic disorder, as well as your individual risk of passing a particular disorder on to your children, will be explained to you. You may also want to talk about the effect an inherited disorder may have on your child's quality of life; and how that disorder could be treated afterwards.

You may be offered genetic counselling if there is any condition within your own personal medical history, or the medical history of your partner or either of your families, that could suggest a risk. Genetic counselling may also be offered to older women, particularly those over 40, whose babies are statistically more prone to chromosomal disorders. Couples who are first cousins may be offered counselling, because they share a greater proportion of the same genes (inherited from their mutual grandparents) so there is more chance of any hereditary disorder being passed on.

Sometimes, entire communities are at greater risk of specific disorders. These are groups that, historically,

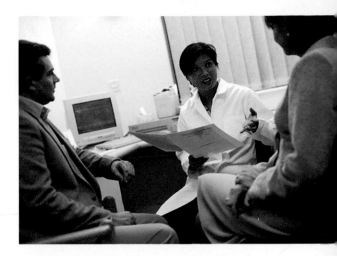

A genetic counsellor will help you and your partner to interpret scans and test results, in the context of your two families' histories. You will be given probabilities rather than forecasts; genetics cannot predict the future.

tend to intermarry for strong cultural or religious reasons, with the result that all the families in the group are genetically related to each other.

The genetic consequence of this is that the gene pool is smaller, and this has the effect of increasing the chance that any disorder that may exist will become more widely distributed than usual within the community. This increased risk will persist even after the cultural circumstances that created it have changed. So, for example, Ashkenazi Jews are more at risk than other people of Tay-Sachs disease. People of Mediterranean or Asian origin are statistically more likely to inherit thalassaemia.

GENETICS AND PROBABILITY

On its own, the fact that there is an inherited disorder in your family does not mean that you are a carrier of the disease, nor that you will inevitably pass it on to the next generation. Remember, only half your genes come from each parent, so there is only a 50:50 chance of any single gene being passed from a parent to you, or from you to your child. Moreover, the mere presence of a gene in your genetic make-up does not of itself mean that you will display that characteristic: not all genes are active in every person or every generation.

In the case of some hereditary diseases, you can be tested to determine whether or not you or your partner is a carrier. This is done by means of a blood test. You cannot be given a simple yes or no answer to the question 'Will my child develop a hereditary disease?'. All that can be determined is a statistical probability, and this can be used to advise you.

Relaxation and fertility

Stress and anxiety can delay conception, so it is important that you incorporate plenty of rest and relaxation into your life when you are trying to conceive. Exercise, too, is an essential part of your preconceptual care. Moderate physical activity not only contributes to general good health, but it also relieves stress and tension, thus helping to keep your hormones and menstrual cycle functioning normally.

EXERCISE

Incorporate three or four exercise sessions of about 30 minutes into every week. Walking in the fresh air and swimming are good options for women who are pregnant or hoping to become so, because they can be done for long periods without causing excessive tiredness. Whichever activity you choose, avoid exhausting yourself. Make sure that you combine your fitness programme with a healthy diet and drinking plenty of water.

SLEEP

How much sleep we need varies depending on our age, health and particular constitution. Most adults need about eight to ten hours a night in order to feel fully rested. Good-quality regular sleep is an absolute must for good health. As we sleep, our blood pressure decreases. The

> **❝ Exercise can relieve stress and tension, thus helping to keep your hormones and menstrual cycle functioning normally. ❞**

body's repair systems work more quickly and efficiently, so sleep is the time when damage is repaired. In addition, the body's natural elimination systems (the liver, the kidneys and the circulation) can carry out their work without having to process additional toxins from the air outside or from the food that we eat.

To help ensure a good night's rest, try the following:

- Establish a good sleep routine. Go to bed and get up at roughly the same time each day, even if you have had a bad night.
- Eat your last meal of the day at least three hours before bedtime. You can have a small snack before bed if necessary.
- Avoid stimulants in the evening, such as tea, coffee, alcohol and nicotine. Having a milky drink before bed can help you to get to sleep.
- Make sure the bedroom is well ventilated – open the window a little at night.
- Clear any daytime clutter, such as a computer, TV, newspapers or work papers, from the bedroom. If you can't clear them away, cover them up with a throw.
- Make sure that your bed gives you good support without being too hard.
- Avoid having stimulating discussions or arguments before bedtime – put them off until the next day.
- If you can't sleep, get up and go into another room. Try again in a few minutes or when you feel sleepy.

ACHIEVING PEACE OF MIND

Relaxation and peace of mind are important elements of your preconceptual care. Some psychologists say that there are three basic elements of happiness: having a good relationship, having something to do and having something to look forward to. Those are three important goals to work towards, but, whatever your circumstances, you can develop a relaxed attitude.

One step to peace of mind is to look at your present problems, worries and dilemmas. If you feel anxious

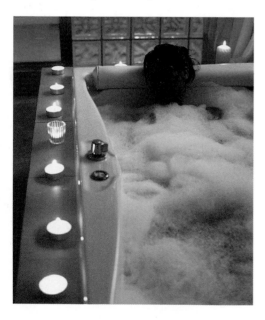

Relaxation is an important aspect of improving your fertility. An aromatherapy bath, with candles, can be a wonderful way to release the strains of the day.

about any area of your life, sit down and write a list of the issues that worry you. Put them into categories: practical, financial, emotional, family and so on.

Now consider how you may be able to deal with those worries. Nagging long-term problems can be both destructive and extremely fatiguing: it is much better to deal with them if you are able to, or at least try and adopt a more relaxed attitude towards them. If you feel overwhelmed by a particular problem, it may be worth getting some additional help from either a complementary therapist or a counsellor.

Assess your priorities and take steps to deal with them in order of importance. List problems, too, so that you can seek help if necessary to resolve them.

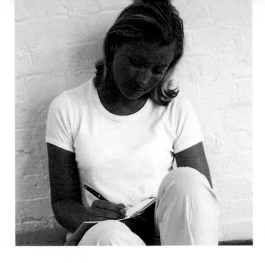

MONITOR YOUR STRESS RATING

Everybody has some stress in their life. However, it is possible to put a figure on your stress levels, as shown in this test devised by Holmes and Rahe in 1967.

Tick those events you have experienced in the last year, then add up your total. This will give an indication of the source and degree of stress in your life.

EVENT	SCORE
☐ Death of spouse	100
☐ Divorce	73
☐ Marital separation	65
☐ Prison term	63
☐ Death of a close family member	63
☐ Personal injury or illness	53
☐ Marriage	50
☐ Loss of job	47
☐ Marital reconciliation	45
☐ Retirement	45
☐ Change in family member's health	44
☐ Pregnancy	40
☐ Sex difficulties	39
☐ Addition to family	39
☐ Business readjustment	39
☐ Change in financial state	38
☐ Death of a close friend	37
☐ Change to different type of work	36
☐ More or fewer marital arguments	35
☐ Taking out a large mortgage or loan	31
☐ Foreclosure on mortgage or loan	30
☐ Change in work responsibilities	29
☐ Son or daughter leaving home	29
☐ Trouble with in-laws	29
☐ Outstanding personal achievement	28
☐ Spouse begins or stops work	26
☐ Starting or finishing school	26
☐ Change in living conditions	25
☐ Change of personal habits	24
☐ Trouble with boss	23
☐ Change in work hours or conditions	20

EVENT	SCORE
☐ Change in residence	20
☐ Change in school	20
☐ Change in recreational habits	19
☐ Change in church activities	19
☐ Change in social activities	18
☐ Taking out a small mortgage/loan	17
☐ Change in sleeping habits	16
☐ More or fewer family gatherings	15
☐ Change in eating habits	15
☐ Holiday	13
☐ Christmas	12
☐ Minor violation of the law	11

TOTAL SCORE

Assess your stress rating by adding up the figures for each life event that you have experienced. If your total comes to less than 150, your rating is normal. If your rating comes to 150–299, you are experiencing more stressful events than the average person. A high level of stress can undermine your chances of getting pregnant, and you may be at risk of developing a stress-related condition. A score of 300 or more is very high, and your risk of becoming ill is much greater than normal.

If you have a high stress rating – or if you are feeling anxious, stressed or overwhelmed – make sure that you dedicate time each day to de-stressing and relaxing. There are many ways to do this – what is important is to find one that works for you. For example, you may need to do more exercise, take up yoga or meditation, or simply incorporate some 'me-time' into your day.

Preconception yoga stretches

Many doctors recommend yoga exercises such as these as an effective way to relax, which may help those trying to conceive. These exercises also increase blood flow (and so the supply of oxygen and nutrients and removal of accumulated waste products, which may cause imbalances), flexibility and strength in areas vital to conception, pregnancy and birth – the pelvic region, hips, abdomen and spine. Many yoga instructors believe that this approach encourages energy to flow freely around the body in a way that makes it more open to conception.

Pelvic movements with focused awareness

These relaxing movements encourage increased awareness, blood flow and flexibility in the pelvic area.

Feel that you are opening up to new healing energy and letting go of any tension there.

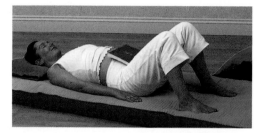

1 Lie down, with a large book and three cushions beside you. Place one cushion under your head and tuck in your chin to lengthen the neck. Bend your knees and plant the feet hip-width apart on the floor. Place the book on your lower abdomen, so that it is evenly balanced on the hip and pubic bones. Place your arms alongside your body, with palms facing down to support you. As you breathe in, press on your hands and arch your lower back so that the navel and hip bones rise and your pelvis (and the book) tips towards your feet.

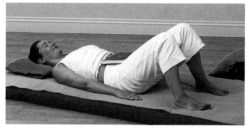

2 As you breathe out, gently pull in the navel towards the spine and press on your hands to lift the sitting bone (coccyx) just off the floor. With this movement, the pelvis (and the book) is now tipped backwards, towards your head. Keep your waist against the floor and move the lower spine only. Repeat these two movements several times. As you do so, bring real awareness of thought to your body. This will help you to do the movements in a focused way. Breathe naturally as you work; do not hold your breath.

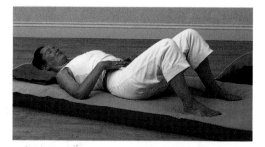

3 Now place your hands, in a relaxed pose, on top of the book. Breathe deeply, bringing your awareness to the pelvic region. Feel the movements of the book over the pelvic area as you breathe in and out slowly for several minutes.

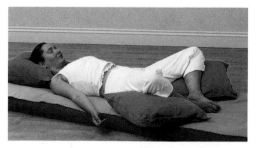

4 Remove the book and bring the soles of your feet together so that your knees fall outward. Support them with the remaining two cushions. Place your hands, palms up, beside you in a gesture of openness and complete surrender. Relax for several minutes.

Improving flexibility and muscle tone in the lower body

These three simple exercises improve flexibility in the spine and hips and strengthen the abdominal muscles. Work gently at first; your strength and flexibility will improve with practice. Relax afterwards and feel the effect of the exercises on your muscles and breath. Keep your coccyx on the floor throughout.

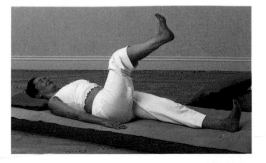

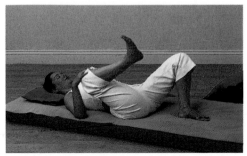

1 Lie on your back with a cushion under your head and your arms, palms down, alongside your body. Bend your right leg, keeping the left leg stretched with the ankle flexed. Make large cycling circles with your right leg until you feel tired. Then rest for a few moments with both legs stretched out – be aware of the muscles in the right side of the lower abdomen. Repeat the same number of circles with your left leg, and then rest again.

2 With your left knee bent and your left foot planted firmly on the floor, take hold of your right knee and move the right leg in circles from the hip. This releases any tightness in the groin and hip joint. Keep breathing naturally and work very gently, especially if the area feels stiff. It doesn't matter if the movements are very small, since your flexibility will gradually improve. Rest, then repeat the movements on the other side.

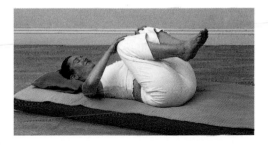

3 Now work with both knees and the breath. Breathe in as you take the knees out to the sides. Breathe out as you pull your knees close to your chest to stretch your lower back. Again, work very gently and build up your ability slowly – in yoga the point is always to work with the body, not to force it into uncomfortable positions. Repeat several times, then rest.

Lying twist

This powerful but simple twisting exercise opens up and relaxes both the shoulders and the hips. This in turn helps to make the entire spine more flexible, creating space between the vertebrae.

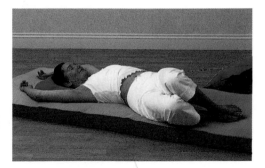

Lie down, raise your arms, bend them at the elbows, and place them on the floor above or beside your head. This position opens and lifts the chest. Bend your knees and place your feet together on the floor. Breathe in. As you breathe out, lower both knees to the right, ensuring that you keep them together. The aim is to place your right knee on the floor without letting your left elbow leave the floor, but only take it as far as feels comfortable. As you breathe in, raise your knees to the centre, still keeping them pressed together. As you breathe out, lower them to the left and raise them again as you breathe in. Repeat several times, then relax for several minutes,

Common Qs and As

Q: I had a pregnancy terminated when I was 17 – I am now 29 and married and wish to have my first baby. But I am worried that I may not be able to conceive because of the termination.

A: There is probably no reason for you to worry: many women have had a termination – even several terminations – and then gone on to have a healthy baby later on. The best advice is to go ahead and start trying, although you may wish to visit your family doctor to discuss your particular medical history.

Q: I have had thrush and a number of other infections in the past and wonder if this will affect my chances of becoming pregnant.

A: Many women suffer from regular thrush, and there is no reason why this should stop you from conceiving. However, a sexual health check is recommended for all women before attempting to conceive. Explain your circumstances to your family doctor and make sure that you have the full range of checks – especially the one for chlamydia, which often has no symptoms but frequently causes infertility.

Q: I have had two miscarriages early on in my pregnancies. I am now trying to conceive for the third time. Is it likely to happen again?

A: Miscarriage is very distressing, and it is not surprising that you are anxious about conceiving again. However, you may find it reassuring to know that having two successive miscarriages is quite common – you have only a slightly higher than normal risk of having another one. Doctors do not consider that you have a problem until you have had three successive miscarriages.

Get plenty of support before and after conception. If using natural therapies, choose a practitioner who is experienced in treating pregnant women.

Q: How do you know if you have one of the risk factors for pregnancy?

A: Most risk factors cause unusual symptoms. If you notice anything worrying, you should see your family doctor so that any problem can be identified and treated.

Some conditions, however, cause few or no distinctive symptoms. These include fibroids and ovarian cancer. If you are aware of any conditions that have affected members of your family, you should tell your doctor. He or she may recommend a specialist check-up before you try to become pregnant.

Q: We are always so busy, we are often too tired to make love, but I desperately want to have a baby.

A: So, something has to give. Take a look at your daily routine and your weekly schedule – both your own and your partner's – and decide what you can edge out in order to make more time for you and your partner. Beware leaving it too late: if you should encounter problems in conceiving, you may need additional months (or more) for these to be resolved.

You might find it helpful to make a list of all the things you have to do. Put them in order of priority to you. Now see whether you can leave any undone – if so, delete them. Think whether any can be delegated to other people – and do so. Then set yourself a reasonable timescale in which to achieve the rest.

Q: We want to start a family but I am terrified when I read about all the things that can go wrong.

A: Remind yourself that 97 per cent of all pregnancies result in the safe and successful delivery of a normal and healthy baby. With today's antenatal care (which represents preventative health care at its best), problems can be detected and resolved. You really have no reason to be terrified. Starting a family is one of life's great adventures.

Q: We want to start a family but I am scared of the pain of birth.

A: There is now a wide range of pain relief options for labour and delivery. You will be able to tell those responsible for your care that you want maximum pain relief and make sure that that statement is entered on your hospital birth plan. You may also want to consider a water birth, which is thought to reduce the pain. At this stage, it is a good idea for you to confide in your partner and perhaps an additional friend or relative as well.

You may wish to discuss with them who you would like to be with you for the labour and delivery. You could, for example, have your partner as well as your mother or sister or good friend. You may wish to have an acupuncturist or hypnotist with you as well as – or instead of – your partner or relative. It would also be a good idea for your partner to accompany you to antenatal checks and, of course, to the antenatal (parent craft) classes as well.

On the issue of fearing the pain and discomfort of childbirth, there is another reason for you to act now and not delay conceiving. This is because, the younger you are when you give birth, the easier it is likely to be for you. As you get older, your energy levels become lower and your muscles and joints grow weaker and less flexible.

Q: I have read that Pilates and yoga are particularly helpful for both conception and pregnancy. Why is this?

A: Pilates is a system of conditioning exercise that focuses on low impact and relaxing routines. In essence it consists of a series of controlled movements performed within the frame of your body so that no movement will pull you from the centre of your body. Yoga also teaches you to focus, balance and 'centre' both your mind and body. Relaxing Pilates and yoga routines are especially helpful because relief from stress is of vital importance during pregnancy, and when trying to conceive.

If you want to practise Pilates or yoga when you are pregnant, it is important that you start before you conceive, and build up your strength, flexibility and body awareness. Experts say that you should not start Pilates, yoga or any other new form of exercise in the first three months of pregnancy. However, if you already have an established routine, you can usually continue provided that you modify certain positions – a trained yoga or Pilates teacher must advise you on how to do this.

Pilates and yoga also increase the circulation to your growing baby rather than diverting blood from it like other exercises. They develop your overall muscle strength and also increase your flexibility. This helps to prevent lower back pain during pregnancy and also improves your balance. Because Pilates and yoga help you to relax and teach you to breathe deeply and evenly, delivery may prove easier. These forms of exercise can also strengthen the abdominal muscles, making it easier for you to recover from childbirth and regain your pre-pregnancy fitness.

Women who are overweight may find Pilates and yoga particularly useful means of starting to exercise. Having improved their muscle strength and flexibility, they can then progress more easily to regular walking and swimming regimes.

CHAPTER FOUR
Delayed conception

“ Professional help often resolves the problem, leading to a successful pregnancy. ”

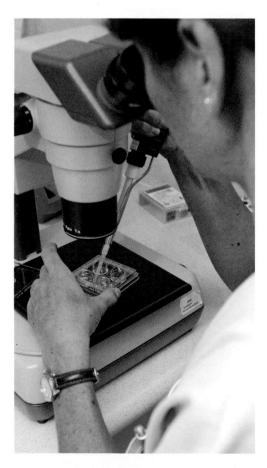

If you and your partner experience a delay in conceiving, remember first and foremost that this is nothing unusual. For especially long delays, professional help often resolves the problem, leading to a successful pregnancy.

Many people immediately think of IVF (in-vitro fertilization) as the solution to infertility, but this is very much a last-resort solution with a fairly low success rate. Infertility can be caused by all kinds of different problems, outlined in the following pages, and some of these can be resolved relatively simply.

The first step is for both partners to consult the family doctor and ask for a referral to a specialist. In the meantime, the chances of becoming pregnant will be enhanced by both partners doing everything they can to improve their general health and fitness. This means of course giving up smoking, cutting out alcohol, eating healthily and exercising regularly. Relaxation is also a prime consideration. It can be

All kinds of tests and investigations can be undertaken to understand infertility, so do not worry needlessly without seeking medical advice.

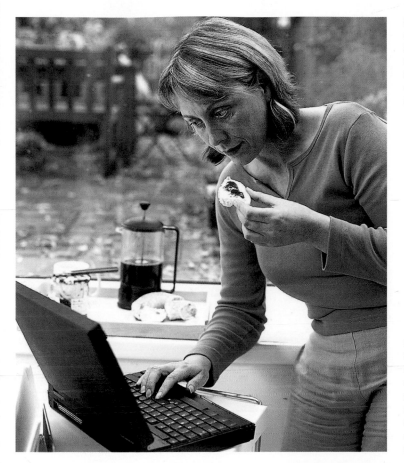

Many people believe that a stressful modern lifestyle, trying to juggle too many tasks and not taking time out for ourselves, contributes to infertility problems.

Meditation is the perfect way to relax and cope with the anxieties that may accompany infertility problems. The simplest form of meditation is simply to focus on gazing at an object such as a flower or crystal.

difficult to maintain a happy, balanced attitude to life while trying to deal with your feelings about delayed conception. However, do whatever you can to relax and have fun with your partner by focusing on those things that you normally enjoy together. Choose activities that you enjoy out of the home to try and take the focus off lovemaking.

About one-third of infertility problems are caused by the woman's reproductive system, one-third by the man's and one-third may be unexplained. Once the problem is found, relatively simple surgery may be the answer. Even unexplained infertility often gives way to unexplained fertility after a period of time. There are lots of good reasons to feel hopeful.

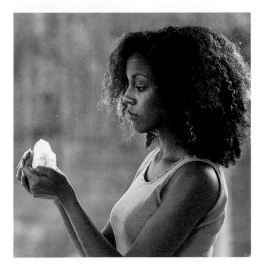

Problems with conceiving

Many couples naturally start to worry if conception does not happen within the first two or three months of trying for a baby. However, delayed conception is extremely common and there is very often no need for a couple to feel anxious.

The months of trying to get pregnant can be an extremely stressful time for both partners. It is all too easy to allow your thoughts to be dominated completely by your desire to have a baby, and to become increasingly worried when conception does not occur. Unfortunately, anxiety can become part of the problem and delay conception still further.

SEEKING MEDICAL HELP

You should see your family doctor if you have been having regular, unprotected sex for a year or longer but have not conceived. Your doctor may check that you are making love at the correct time, and will also ask about your general health and lifestyle – in particular whether you smoke or drink. He or she may also carry out some preliminary tests to rule out some of the obvious causes of infertility.

If these tests do not provide answers, ask to be referred to a consultant gynaecologist. It is very important that both partners attend all these consultations – because the problem may be with either partner or, sometimes, with both of you. In one-third of cases, failure or delay in conceiving arises from the woman's reproductive system; in another third there is a problem with the man's reproductive system; in the remaining third the problem lies with both partners or its cause simply cannot be identified. A gynaecologist will take a detailed medical history and will also check lifestyle factors that could be the reason for

> **"Delayed conception is extremely common and there is very often no need for a couple to feel anxious."**

delayed conception. Various checks may be done on your blood and on the man's blood and semen. The reproductive organs of both partners are likely to be checked for damage, blockages and other problems.

These investigations may be invasive and time-consuming. However, they and any subsequent treatment can be very fruitful: up to 40 per cent of couples who seek specialist help achieve a pregnancy within two years. The major causes of infertility, together with their treatments, are discussed on the pages that follow.

MISCARRIAGE

In some cases, the woman may actually have conceived, but she may have had a miscarriage without realizing it. A high proportion of miscarriages occur within the first two months of pregnancy, often before the woman knows that she is pregnant. The loss of a baby through early miscarriage is much more common than many people believe, and may account for many cases of what is thought to be delayed conception. It could be that as many as over half of all early pregnancies end in miscarriage.

The warning signs for an impending miscarriage include vaginal bleeding, abdominal cramps and backache similar to those of a period. Excessive vomiting can also be a symptom. Once a miscarriage starts, there is little that can be done to halt it. However, it is important that you seek medical advice immediately because there is a risk of infection and complications.

INVESTIGATING MISCARRIAGE

Having a miscarriage can be a very traumatic experience. For some women it is just as distressing as a bereavement, even when it occurs in the early stages of pregnancy. It may be of some comfort to know that miscarriage, particularly in the early months, is very common. It does not mean that there is anything inherently wrong with you, or that you are likely to miscarry next time you become pregnant. The vast majority of women go on to have successful pregnancies after experiencing a miscarriage. For this reason, having one or even two early miscarriages is not usually seen as a reason for medical investigation.

WORKING TOGETHER
Trying for a baby can involve many moments of both expectation and disappointment. It is difficult to cope with a specific problem with conception, but also hard to bear a failure to conceive where the cause simply cannot be identified. It is extremely important that you both find ways to relax as much as you can and to enjoy your relationship fully, so that trying for a baby does not become a negative and unhappy experience.

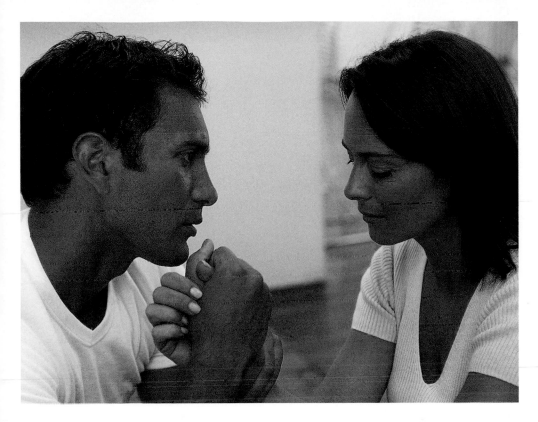

Tests are usually done if a woman experiences repeated miscarriages: this is defined as three or more successive miscarriages with no successful pregnancy occurring in between. After suffering three miscarriages, you should seek specialist help and advice. A late miscarriage – one that occurs after 14 weeks – should also be investigated.

Your family doctor will be able to refer you to a consultant gynaecologist if you have had recurrent miscarriages. In some cases, couples may then be referred to a genetic counsellor. Genetic counselling may help to determine the level or risk of future pregnancies, and to discuss the best way forwards.

WHY MISCARRIAGE HAPPENS

Doctors do not know why so many pregnancies end unsuccessfully, and determining the cause of a miscarriage can be very difficult or even impossible. Some of the known causes of early miscarriage include:

- A major abnormality in the baby. About three in every five early miscarriages are thought to be connected to fetal abnormality.
- The mother contracting rubella, listeriosis or chlamydia during the pregnancy.

It can be very distressing for both partners when pregnancy does not happen straight away, especially if you have delayed having a baby. It is essential to be totally supportive of each other.

- The failure of the fertilized egg to implant successfully in the lining of the uterus.
- The mother having a low level of progesterone, which is needed to sustain the pregnancy.

Later miscarriage (after 14 weeks) can be the result of:
- An abnormality in the uterus, such as a large fibroid.
- A weak (incompetent) cervix. This is a condition in which the cervix dilates instead of remaining tightly closed during pregnancy.
- Certain antenatal tests; amniocentesis, for example, carries a 1 in 200 risk of miscarriage.
- The mother having diabetes, epilepsy, asthma, kidney disease or high blood pressure.

Miscarriages are more common in very young women or women over 35. Many people think that minor injuries or distress can cause a miscarriage, but there is no medical evidence to support this.

WOMEN'S REPRODUCTIVE PROBLEMS

The conditions listed below include the most common reasons for female infertility. However, that is not to say that all women affected by them necessarily become infertile – some women with small fibroids, say, may have successful pregnancies without treatment. Treatment is an option in the case of most disorders.

Polycystic ovaries

This is a common condition in which many small cysts form in the ovaries. Polycystic ovary syndrome affects about one in ten women. Some of these women will encounter a variety of hormone-related problems, including infertility.

Women with polycystic ovaries may have no symptoms – with the result that they only know that they have the condition when fertility tests are done. However, symptoms can include:
- Obesity.
- Excessive hair growth on the face or body.
- Acne.
- Infrequent or no menstrual periods.
- Male-pattern baldness (the form of hair loss that is most commonly found in males – namely, losing hair first from the temples and then from the crown, with the bald area on the crown gradually widening).

Drug treatment is sometimes used to induce ovulation in women with polycystic ovaries. Otherwise, the cysts may be treated by being cauterized with a needle. This procedure is done by laparoscopy, in which a fibre-optic tube is inserted into the pelvic area through a small incision made just below the navel. This enables doctors to examine the woman's reproductive organs, take samples and carry out some minor surgery. A general anaesthetic is given.

Endometriosis

One in ten of all women referred for fertility testing turns out to be affected by endometriosis, making it a major cause of infertility. In this condition, cells similar to those of the lining of the uterus (the endometrium) become established outside it. They can grow anywhere in the pelvic area – for example, on the ovaries, in the Fallopian tubes, bladder, uterus, bowel, peritoneum or on the pelvic wall.

These stray endometrial cells respond to natural changes in hormone levels in the same way as those inside the uterus. That is, they increase during part of the month and break down when the lining is being shed (the period). However, because these cells are trapped inside the pelvic area, they cannot leave the body. Instead, they become inflamed and cause adhesions, which can cause one internal organ to become stuck to another. They may also form swellings which fill with dark blood – chocolate cysts.

ENDOMETRIOSIS

If you suffer with severe back ache, abdominal pain or strong cramps during menstruation, ask your doctor to refer you for a specialist check for endometriosis. In this condition, cells like those of the uterus lining grow elsewhere in the pelvis, in the areas shown below.

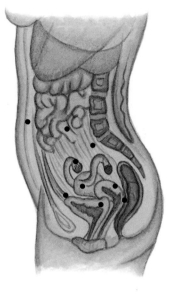

Possible endometriosis sites include: abdominal wall, intestines, Fallopian tubes, ovaries, appendix, uterus, peritoneum (lining of abdomen), cervix, rectum, bladder and vulva.

Many women who are affected by endometriosis think that they merely have painful periods, with the result that the condition often goes undetected for a long time – until fertility testing starts, in fact. The symptoms of endometriosis can include severe backache, abdominal pain and cramps during periods, and pain at ovulation, during bowel movements and during sex. The woman may sometimes also experience nausea and dizziness. Endometriosis is diagnosed by close examination of the pelvis, using a laparoscope.

The condition is usually treated by hormone therapy or by surgery. The procedure known as thermal coagulator treatment uses helium gas ionized by an electric current to dry out the endometrial cells. This procedure has had good results, and its other advantage is that it can be performed quickly.

Pelvic inflammatory disease (PID)

Infection can often cause inflammation in the uterus, Fallopian tubes and ovaries – a condition known as pelvic inflammatory disease. This is a common cause of infertility and other pregnancy-related complications. It is estimated that women who have suffered with PID have a seven-fold risk of ectopic pregnancy.

The bacteria that cause gonorrhoea and chlamydia are thought to be the main causes of PID, although bacteria that normally exist harmlessly in the bowel or gut may also be the culprit. The bacteria enter the body through the vagina and then work up through the cervix into the pelvic cavity. The infection may occur as a consequence of sexually transmitted chlamydia, childbirth, miscarriage, termination or the fitting of an IUD.

In some cases, PID causes no symptoms other than the woman's inability to become pregnant. It is therefore often not detected until fertility testing starts. The condition is also sometimes misdiagnosed as either endometriosis or appendicitis because it can cause similar symptoms. Where symptoms occur, they can include abdominal pain, exhaustion, high temperatures and very heavy, painful periods. The pain has been described as a dull ache across the lower abdomen. In some cases, it may be so intense that the woman is unable to move. The scar tissue caused by PID can increase the risk of recurrent infection and it can cause pain during sex.

PID is diagnosed by means of an internal examination and a laparoscopy. It is usually treated with antibiotics. In severe cases, the woman may need to be admitted to hospital so that antibiotics can be given to her intravenously (directly into the veins).

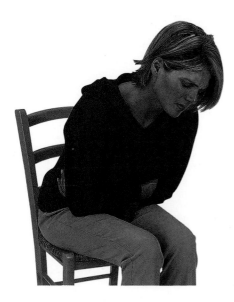

ECTOPIC PREGNANCY

Sometimes a pregnancy can start to develop in the Fallopian tubes rather than in the uterus. An ectopic pregnancy is normally accompanied by severe abdominal pain, and the woman will need emergency treatment to remove the pregnancy.

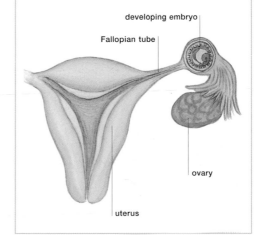

developing embryo

Fallopian tube

ovary

uterus

Ectopic pregnancy

An ectopic pregnancy is one that starts to develop in one of the Fallopian tubes or, more rarely, in another site in the abdominal cavity rather than in the uterus. It can cause permanent damage to the tube, leading to infertility. Doctors do not know why an ectopic pregnancy occurs. However, it is more common if the Fallopian tube has already been damaged by infection, surgery or by a previous ectopic pregnancy.

An ectopic pregnancy can be extremely serious, even life-threatening, and so the woman must get immediate medical treatment. The symptoms can include intense pain in the abdominal area and vaginal bleeding. Ectopic pregnancies are sometimes initially diagnosed as appendicitis or miscarriage.

An ectopic pregnancy cannot develop normally. Once an ectopic pregnancy is confirmed, surgery is needed to remove it. Sometimes, part of the Fallopian tube and part of the ovary may have to be removed as well, although doctors will avoid this whenever possible. Women who have suffered one ectopic pregnancy are at a higher risk of experiencing another one. However, many women who have had an ectopic pregnancy go on to have a perfectly healthy pregnancy.

Many women suffer menstrual cramps. However, severe abdominal pain should always be investigated. It may be a sign of one of several serious conditions.

Polyps and fibroids

Different forms of benign (non-cancerous) tumours or growths, polyps and fibroids can cause infertility in women. Doctors do not know why these grow.

Polyps have a stalk by which they attach themselves to the membrane lining the cervix or uterus. They may cause no symptoms, or the woman may experience a watery discharge streaked with blood between her periods and after intercourse.

Fibroids are bundles of muscle fibres that develop in the muscular wall of the uterus. They can vary in size from a small marble to a large ball. Fibroids are very common – one in five women over the age of 30 develops them. Like polyps, they may cause no symptoms. Where symptoms do occur, they may include long-lasting periods and heavy menstrual bleeding, including flooding and passing clots. The woman may also develop anaemia because of the excessive blood loss, which can then lead to feelings of exhaustion, breathlessness and depression. Other symptoms include severe cramps, incontinence, constipation and cystitis.

Polyps and fibroids are diagnosed by internal examination, ultrasound scan or laparoscopy. The woman may also be given a hysteroscopy, in which a viewing instrument is passed up the vagina into the uterus, or she may be offered a hysterosalpingogram, in which a dye is injected through the cervix so that X-rays of the reproductive organs can be taken. Polyps and fibroids are usually removed surgically. Drug treatment may be recommended to shrink large fibroids before surgery.

Early menopause

The menopause usually starts in the woman's late forties but some women may stop having periods in their thirties or even in their twenties. Women affected may at first think that they are pregnant. However, as well as the periods stopping, other symptoms can include hot flushes, night sweats, insomnia, vaginal drying, painful intercourse, loss of libido, genito-urinary infections, thinning of the skin, splitting of the nails, aches and pains, and incontinence. Women may also experience mood changes, anxiety, irritability, poor memory and poor concentration as well as subsequent loss of confidence.

If a doctor suspects premature menopause, the woman will be referred for a laparoscopy. In this procedure, the ovaries are examined by a laparoscope (a fibre-optic tube); this allows the doctor to see if the woman's ovaries contain follicles with eggs. Women who experience premature menopause may still achieve a pregnancy, but only through assisted conception.

Incompatibility

Failure to conceive may be due to an incompatibility between a man's sperm and a woman's cervical mucus. In these cases, the mucus contains antibodies that destroy the man's sperm before it can reach the egg. A post-coital test may be needed in which a sample of fluid is taken from the woman's cervix six to thirty-six hours after intercourse. This may be treated with drugs or the man's semen may be injected into the woman's uterus to avoid contact with the cervix. Assisted conception may also be an option.

INFERTILITY IN MEN

The reason for male infertility is usually defective sperm or a problem with delivering the sperm to the woman's vagina. It is rare for there to be no sperm at all. Usually the problem is that not enough sperm are being produced or that they are not strong enough to make the journey.

Abnormal sperm production

Sperm may be defective in:
- Quantity – if there are fewer than 20 million sperm per millilitre of ejaculate, the sperm count is said to be low.
- Motility – at least 40 per cent of the sperm should be moving in a healthy sample.
- Normality – the sperm should not be deformed.

If you are having difficulty conceiving, the man's semen will be analysed under a microscope for numbers of

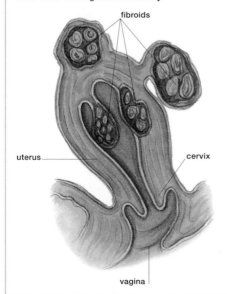

FIBROIDS

These are bundles of muscle that have grown in the muscular wall of the uterus. They can delay or prevent conception, so early treatment is essential for women wishing to have a family.

fibroids

uterus

cervix

vagina

sperm, motility, normality, infection and antibodies. The temperature of the testicles may be assessed by thermography. Some experts maintain that temperature is a defining factor in fertility, while many others disagree.

The man will also be screened for a number of diseases such as diabetes and kidney disease, for example, which can affect sperm production. Other male fertility tests include testicular biopsy and testicular X-ray in case of a genetic problem or childhood disease such as mumps, which may have led to problems with the sperm. Often the cause of low sperm count cannot be identified, and so it cannot be treated. In some cases, therefore, assisted conception may be recommended.

Sperm delivery problems

There can be problems that stop the sperm from reaching the vagina. The major one is impotence, but another cause may be damage to the man's reproductive tubes, which may be due to a sexually transmitted disease or to some other cause.

Some cases of impotence and erectile problems may be treated by medication such as Viagra. Counselling may be offered if the impotence is thought to have a psychological cause. More often, however, male impotence is associated with a physical problem. Some of these conditions can be quite serious – they include heart disease, narrowing of the arteries, diabetes and high blood pressure – so it is important that men suffering from impotence should see their doctor. If the cause of the impotence is not treatable, artificial insemination may be an option.

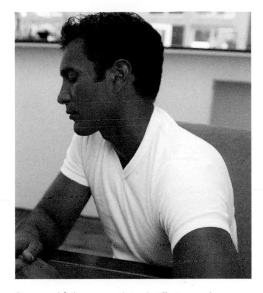

Stress and fatigue may adversely affect a man's sperm count and the quality of the sperm he produces, as well as diminishing his desire to make love.

Damage to the tubes that transport sperm – the epididymis or vas deferens – may be remedied by microsurgery. If the man has had a vasectomy, this can be reversed. However, the chances of this reversal procedure being successful are relatively low.

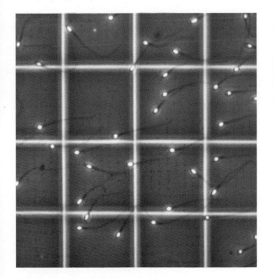

This shows human sperm occurring in a normal quantity – at least 30 million sperm per millilitre ejaculate. The lines on the screen assist counting.

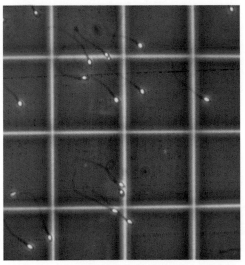

By comparison, this sample shows a low sperm count of under 20 million sperm. A temporary low count may be caused by excess alcohol, smoking, stress or illness.

Fertility treatment

Many couples who have sought professional help with conception go on to have a child naturally. Others may learn that the cause of the infertility cannot be treated or that it cannot be explained. In these cases, assisted conception may be an option. It should be remembered that infertility investigations and treatments can take a great deal of time, and they can also be very intrusive. It is important that both partners take steps to care for themselves and to support each other during what can be a difficult time.

SEEING A SPECIALIST

Various tests need to be done before a decision is made to start fertility treatment. Your family doctor may carry out some preliminary investigations. These tests may uncover a simple problem that the doctor can treat. If not, you should be referred to a specialist for further investigation.

A specialist will want to ensure that the woman is ovulating, the man is producing healthy sperm in sufficient quantities and that the sperm and egg are able to meet. The specialist will investigate the woman's menstrual cycle and ovulatory cycle, the health of her reproductive system and her general health. If the specialist suspects that she is not ovulating, he or she may take blood tests to check her hormone levels at frequent intervals during her menstrual cycle; her ovaries may also be scanned using ultrasound to check when and if ovulation takes place.

The man will be asked to provide two or more samples of semen. These will be analysed under a microscope to check that there is a sufficient quantity of sperm and that they are healthy. If the sperm count is low, the man's testosterone levels may be checked – a lack of this hormone can affect sperm production.

If the woman is ovulating and there is not a problem with the man's sperm, the doctor will carry out further tests to see why sperm and egg are not meeting. A sample of cervical mucus may be collected after the couple have sex and tested to see if there is any obvious incompatibility. The woman's reproductive system may be examined by laparoscopy to detect any blockages or damage, and the man's reproductive organs will also be checked.

Before starting fertility treatment, a specialist will discuss your general health and lifestyle to ensure that these are not factors in any delay in conception. Sometimes you may be given general health advice to carry out before or during treatment, which may include the following guidelines.

Common health advice for men

A specialist may advise:
- Losing weight if overweight.
- Stopping smoking – if you continue to smoke while receiving fertility treatment, it may be less effective.
- Reducing alcohol intake.
- Avoiding caffeine.
- Abstaining from any drugs – cannabis and cocaine, for example, affect sperm quality and quantity.
- Avoiding excessive exercise.
- Having a healthy diet.
- Monitoring the temperature of the testicles – overheating may affect sperm production.
- Reducing stress and getting enough rest.
- Stopping any non-essential medication that may interfere with sperm production.

In general, the man should comply with this advice for about 70 days before the semen analysis takes place. This is the length of time that it takes to produce sperm.

Common health advice for women

A specialist may advise:
- Losing excess weight if overweight.
- Stopping smoking.
- Giving up alcohol for the time being.
- Avoiding caffeine.
- Abstaining from drugs.
- Having a healthy diet.
- Taking regular, moderate exercise.
- Getting enough regular sleep and relaxation.

ROUTINE FERTILITY TREATMENTS

In many cases, the problem is straightforward and treatable. Fertility treatments may include the following:
- Fertility medication to stimulate ovulation.
- Hormone treatment to encourage sperm production.
- Drug treatment with corticosteroids to suppress production of antibodies to the man's sperm.
- Microsurgery – for example, to repair damage to the Fallopian tubes or male reproductive tubes.
- Other surgery – for example, to remove fibroids.

ASSISTED FERTILITY

If the specialist thinks that a couple are unlikely to achieve a pregnancy naturally, he or she may recommend that they start assisted fertility treatment. This treatment may take the form of artificial insemination or one of the other

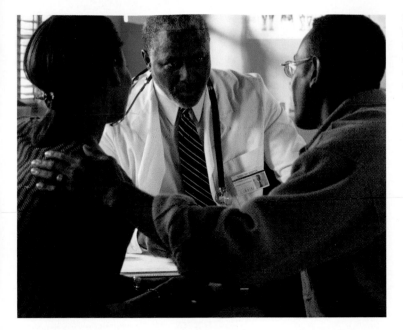

When a couple first consults a fertility specialist, he or she will check their general health and lifestyle before starting investigations.

methods listed below, depending on the cause of the problem. It is extremely important that a couple understand exactly what is involved in any assisted fertility treatment. They need to appreciate its chances of success, and the financial cost that they will need to bear. They will be offered counselling, which is intended to help them to explore their feelings and to be honest with each other about their anxieties and fears.

ARTIFICIAL INSEMINATION

AI, or artificial insemination, involves introducing the partner's sperm into the woman's cervical channel or directly into the uterus when she is ovulating. This is done in hospital, using a syringe. No anaesthetic is necessary for this procedure. Sometimes the semen may be treated in order to remove defective or poor-quality sperm before they are inserted into the woman's body.

Artificial insemination is a useful method for couples in which the woman's body makes antibodies to her partner's sperm, and also for couples who experience sexual difficulties such as impotence or premature ejaculation, low sperm count or blockages in the male reproductive organs. It is sometimes used for cases of unexplained infertility.

DONOR INSEMINATION

Sometimes a donor's sperm may be used instead of that of a male partner. This is known as donor insemination (DI). The method can be used in cases of impotence or defective sperm, as well as by single and lesbian women who wish to have a child.

❝ In many cases, the problem is straightforward and treatable. ❞

IN-VITRO FERTILIZATION (IVF)

So-called test-tube babies are a result of this procedure, which involves mixing the woman's eggs with sperm outside her body.

Before IVF is carried out, the woman will take fertility drugs to stimulate her ovaries into producing more than one egg. The eggs are then collected. One method of doing this involves inserting a laparoscope through a small cut in the abdomen to draw off the egg-producing follicles. This is done under general anaesthetic. Alternatively, a needle is inserted through the abdomen and is then guided with ultrasound to draw off the follicles. This method requires only a local anaesthetic.

The eggs are mixed with sperm in a laboratory and left to incubate for two days at normal body temperature. Provided that both the eggs and the sperm are healthy, 60 per cent of the eggs may be fertilized. A few of the resulting embryos will then be inserted into the uterus via a syringe. No anaesthetic is needed for this procedure. If there are additional eggs that have been fertilized, they may be frozen for future attempts.

The embryos then need to attach themselves to the lining of the uterus – implantation – for a pregnancy to take place. If all the inserted embryos do implant, doctors may recommend removing all but one to give the pregnancy the best chance of success.

When IVF is used

In-vitro fertilization may be used if the man is producing poor-quality sperm, if the woman's body is making antibodies to the sperm, or if she has blocked or scarred Fallopian tubes or irregular ovulation. It is also sometimes recommended for cases of unexplained infertility. IVF can be done using the male partner's or a donor's sperm. Donor eggs can also be used if the woman is not producing her own. In some cases, donor embryos – that is, embryos made from both donor sperm and eggs – may be used.

IVF was successfully used for the first time in 1978, in the UK. It resulted in the birth of the world's first test-tube baby – Louise Brown. Like all assisted conception methods, the success rate of IVF is not high. When two embryos are transferred, there is a one in four (25 per cent) chance of a pregnancy occurring. However, just as pregnancies achieved naturally can end in miscarriage, so too can those that occur as a result of IVF. The percentage of IVF treatments that end in the delivery of a baby is about 15 per cent – in other words, there is a one in seven chance of an IVF treatment resulting in a baby. Most couples who opt for IVF have to go through several treatment cycles.

GAMETE INTRA-FALLOPIAN TRANSFER (GIFT)

GIFT is a variation of IVF that is used when no reason can be found for female infertility, or if the man has a low sperm count. In this procedure, the eggs and sperm are collected as in IVF. Doctors examine the eggs to ensure they are healthy and select up to three for insertion. The eggs are mixed with the sperm, and are then placed immediately in one of the Fallopian tubes, where they are left to fertilize naturally. This procedure is done by laparoscopy, under a general anaesthetic.

GIFT has a success rate of about 25 per cent, which is higher than that of IVF. However, it can be carried out only if the woman's Fallopian tubes are clear.

ZYGOTE INTRA-FALLOPIAN TRANSFER (ZIFT)

This method is very similar to GIFT; the woman's eggs are collected and the eggs mixed with sperm in the same way. However, in this method doctors check that fertilization has taken place before injecting the fused eggs and sperm into the Fallopian tubes.

ZIFT is used when GIFT either hasn't worked or is considered unlikely to work. Again, the woman's Fallopian tubes must be healthy and functioning. The success rate is about 25 per cent. Both GIFT and ZIFT can be done with donor eggs or sperm.

In GIFT, the gynaecologist places selected eggs and sperm in the woman's Fallopian tube, with the aim of fertilization followed by implantation in the uterus.

INTRA-CYTOPLASM SPERM INJECTION (ICSI)

This technique is especially suitable when the man has a low sperm count or produces sperm either of poor quality or low motility. In ICSI, the eggs and sperm are collected in the same way as for IVF. A single sperm is then injected into an egg to ensure that fertilization takes place. The resulting embryo is then placed in the uterus so that implantation can take place. The success rate for each ICSI treatment is about 22 per cent.

DONOR SPERM, EGGS AND EMBRYOS

Sometimes, donated sperm is needed to facilitate a pregnancy. This may be because the male partner may pass on a genetic disease or has a very low sperm count. Donor sperm is also used by lesbian and single women who wish to conceive a child. The donor may be known to the couple. However, more often, the sperm comes from an anonymous donor via a sperm bank.

Another woman's eggs may be used in fertility treatment. The eggs may be fertilized by the male partner's sperm or that of a donor. A few of the resulting embryos are placed in the woman's uterus and she is given hormonal drugs to help maintain the pregnancy. Egg donation is the only assisted conception technique

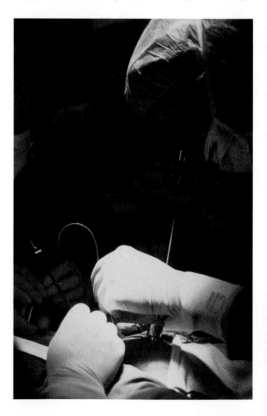

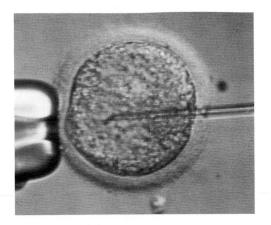

In ICSI, the woman's egg is placed in a dish and injected with a sperm before being transferred to the uterus in the hope of successful implantation.

available for women who are not producing eggs at all, although surrogacy and adoption may be considered. Egg donation may also be used by women who may pass on a genetic disorder to their children.

Egg donation is a complex procedure, requiring the same drug treatment and monitoring as IVF or GIFT. Egg donors are usually women under the age of 35 who have already had their own children. The donor may be a relative or close friend of the couple, or may be anonymous. The use of the technique is limited because of a shortage of donors.

Donor embryos are also used in fertility treatment. They may come from couples who are themselves undergoing fertility treatment and have produced several viable embryos during IVF or other methods. They may also be produced by fertilizing donated eggs with donated sperm. They are used when neither the woman's eggs nor the man's sperm can be used to achieve a healthy pregnancy.

OTHER OPTIONS

Surrogacy and adoption are two options when assisted conception fails. In surrogacy, another woman is used to carry the fertilized egg and give birth to the baby. In some cases, the surrogate conceives using her own egg and the male partner's sperm, and then hands over the baby at birth. Surrogacy can be fraught with legal difficulties, and it works only if all parties are in full agreement about the arrangement and stick to it. Payment is illegal in some countries, including the UK.

Another alternative is adoption. The legal situation surrounding adoption is much clearer than that of surrogacy. However, there are many more couples wanting to adopt a baby than there are babies available. Often, older couples are not eligible for adopting babies.

ACCEPTING THE SITUATION

Some couples may decide to go ahead with fertility treatments, but others may choose not to do so. Still more may call a halt to the treatment after undergoing several unsuccessful attempts. Counselling should always be offered to couples who are undergoing fertility investigations and treatments. It may also be beneficial to seek support from a complementary therapist as well.

It is sometimes the case that a couple who accept their infertility suddenly conceive – much to their joy and surprise. Others come to terms with their infertility, finding other ways to have a fulfilling and happy life.

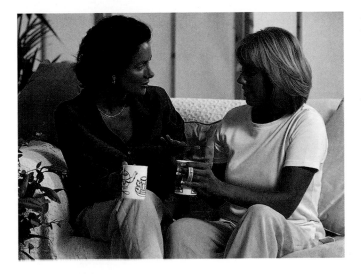

Infertility, which may continue for many years, almost always proves distressing and exhausting. A close friend can be a good source of support. However, be prepared to seek professional counselling via your family doctor if you feel the need to talk through the complex and deeply personal issues involved.

How natural therapies help

Some complementary practitioners believe that therapies may actively assist conception. Most infertility experts and gynaecologists would dispute this. However, there is no doubt that the natural therapies have their part to play in supporting people during the time that they are attempting to conceive.

First and foremost, many complementary therapies, including acupuncture and reflexology, encourage good general health and well-being. They may be useful to those trying to give up smoking and reduce their alcohol consumption, or they may simply help you to feel healthier and more alive, as with the detoxing effects produced by lymphatic massage. Many natural therapies, including massage, aromatherapy, reflexology and yoga, help with relaxation and de-stressing, which can play an important part in conception.

USING THERAPIES FOR EMOTIONAL SUPPORT

Natural therapies, and especially meditation, yoga and relaxation techniques, can be very helpful if you are having difficulty conceiving, allowing you space to express your feelings and come to terms with them. Some people are able to accept the difficulties in becoming pregnant with calm and equanimity, but others are deeply distressed by any delay and need extra support. There is plenty of research and anecdotal evidence to suggest that you are more likely to conceive if you are relaxed, at peace with yourself and able to deal with any negative feelings and anxieties. For example, it is not uncommon for women who have had problems conceiving to get pregnant once

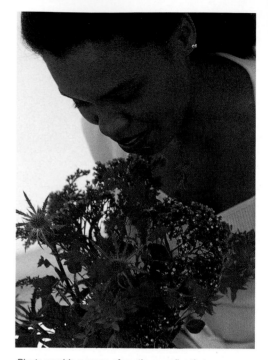

Plants provide a range of gentle remedies that may support conception. For example, certain Bach Flower Remedies aim to promote the kind of relaxed, open state of mind said to increase the chances of falling pregnant.

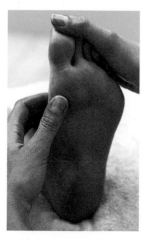

Reflexology can help to boost immunity and energy levels, creating a state of optimum health that is ideal for conception. Always seek medical advice before receiving reflexology during pregnancy (especially within the first three months) or possible pregnancy.

they are on a referral list for specialist advice – the pressure has been taken off them slightly. Negative feelings can all too easily take over. Women who have difficulty conceiving may rapidly find their lives dominated by thoughts of their ovulatory cycle. The start of each month may bring new hope, and the woman may feel determined to ensure that lovemaking coincides with her fertile period. As the time for menstruation approaches, she may become alternately anxious and hopeful, only to feel bitterly disappointed when she knows that she has not conceived. All this can be exhausting and stressful, and her self-esteem may drop.

Having children is seen as a natural process. Many women, in particular, feel very angry when it does not happen for them. It can be particularly hard to accept if they have spent years using contraception so as not to become pregnant at the wrong time or with the wrong partner. At the same time, a woman may start to feel guilty or inadequate. She may look for reasons in her past – wondering, for example, if the delay is somehow due to a previous termination or a past infection. Doctors can often be reassuring on these points.

At the same time, the man may be unhappy about the way his sex life with his partner is dominated by ovulation charts. He may feel taken for granted, wonder if his partner is more interested in having a child than in a happy relationship, and suppress his own feelings about a longed-for conception so that he is able to support the woman. From a conception standpoint, he too may benefit from supportive natural therapies, to improve his general well-being and keep him de-stressed.

Part of the holistic approach to health means that, as well as specific therapies, partners must learn to open up and speak to each other, in order to receive loving support and reassurance from each other. Friends or relatives can also be very helpful, although it is important to remember that not everyone has sufficient understanding and sensitivity in this situation. It can be an excellent idea to seek help from a professional counsellor, who will help you to explore any complex feelings and emotions you may have.

USING AFFIRMATION AND VISUALIZATION

Controlled breathing, meditation, visualization and affirmation work can all help both partners to get into the best mental and physical state to deal with the pre-conception period. Try the following exercise, adapting it to suit your personal situation:

- Choose a place where you will not be interrupted. Sit comfortably, with your back straight, perhaps sitting on a cushion cross-legged, or seated in a chair.
- Take a few deep breaths. Close your eyes. As you breathe, relax your shoulders and your face muscles. Concentrate on your breathing. You can focus on the air passing in and out of your nostrils or the rise and fall of your chest – whichever is easier for you.
- Bring your attention to the centre of your chest, the heart area. Notice how it feels as your breathe in and out – is there tension or pain here? Just notice the feeling, but don't try to change it. If you find focusing difficult, place your hands on your chest, and feel them rise and fall with your breath.
- As you continue to breathe, wish yourself well. There are several ways you can do this: some people like to imagine a pink light in the heart area that slowly expands and grows to encompass their entire body; others like to repeat affirmative phrases in their head. Try the following phrases: "May I be happy, May I be well, May I be safe, May I be at ease in the world". If you prefer, make up your own affirmation.
- Continue for a few minutes. Now visualize your partner in front of you. Imagine the pink light growing

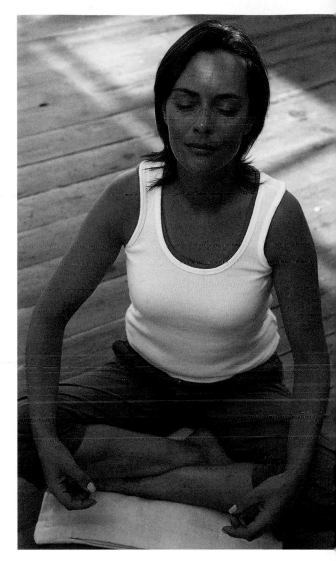

Feel completely free to include whatever elements you wish in pre-conception meditations or visualizations – only you know what feels calming and positive.

to encompass you both, and spend a few moments enjoying its warm loving embrace. If you are using the affirmation technique, turn your good wishes towards your partner: "May you be happy..." etc. After a few minutes, wish both yourself and your partner well: "May we be happy..." etc.
- Now, slowly let the pink light or the words fade away. Bring your attention back to your breathing. Continue sitting quietly for a minute or two, then get up slowly.

How do I know I am pregnant?

Some women believe that they sensed the conception of their babies: they did not need to wait for a missed period or other symptoms to know that they were pregnant. This feeling could simply be intuition, or it is possible that these women are able to detect tiny changes inside the body that are associated with the first secretions of the pregnancy hormones. However, most women cannot be sure that they are pregnant until they have had it confirmed by a pregnancy test.

EARLY SIGNS AND SYMPTOMS

The first definite sign of pregnancy is a missed period, known medically as amenorrhoea. Pregnancy is the most likely reason for a missed period, but it is not the only one – stress is another possible explanation. It is therefore best not to assume that you are pregnant just because you have missed your period. The following signs are other early indicators of pregnancy, some of which may occur before you miss a period. However, many women do not notice them until later in the pregnancy:

- Increased tiredness.
- Feeling nauseous, particularly in the mornings.
- Urinating more frequently than usual.
- Tenderness in the breasts.
- Changes in taste, such as a sudden craving for a particular food or a metallic taste in the mouth.

CONFIRMING A PREGNANCY

Most women do their first pregnancy test at home. Pregnancy-testing kits are available from any pharmacy, and they are very accurate. The tests work by measuring the amount of one of the pregnancy hormones, human chorionic gonadotrophin (HCG), in your urine. If enough HCG is present, it triggers a reaction in the test. This is

WHEN YOUR BABY IS DUE

If you know the date of your last period, you can work out your estimated date of delivery using the chart below. The delivery date is normally 40 weeks from the date of your last period but it can be up to two weeks earlier or later. A delivery outside those dates would be considered premature or post-mature.

MONTH	ESTIMATED DATE OF DELIVERY	MONTH
January	1 2 3 4 5 6 7 8 9 10 11 12 13 14 15 16 17 18 19 20 21 22 23 24 25 26 27 28 29 30 31	January
October	8 9 10 11 12 13 14 15 16 17 18 19 20 21 22 23 24 25 26 27 28 29 30 31 1 2 3 4 5 6 7	November
February	1 2 3 4 5 6 7 8 9 10 11 12 13 14 15 16 17 18 19 20 21 22 23 24 25 26 27 28	February
November	8 9 10 11 12 13 14 15 16 17 18 19 20 21 22 23 24 25 26 27 28 29 30 1 2 3 4 5	December
March	1 2 3 4 5 6 7 8 9 10 11 12 13 14 15 16 17 18 19 20 21 22 23 24 25 26 27 28 29 30 31	March
December	6 7 8 9 10 11 12 13 14 15 16 17 18 19 20 21 22 23 24 25 26 27 28 29 30 31 1 2 3 4 5	January
April	1 2 3 4 5 6 7 8 9 10 11 12 13 14 15 16 17 18 19 20 21 22 23 24 25 26 27 28 29 30	April
January	6 7 8 9 10 11 12 13 14 15 16 17 18 19 20 21 22 23 24 25 26 27 28 29 30 31 1 2 3 4	February
May	1 2 3 4 5 6 7 8 9 10 11 12 13 14 15 16 17 18 19 20 21 22 23 24 25 26 27 28 29 30 31	May
February	5 6 7 8 9 10 11 12 13 14 15 16 17 18 19 20 21 22 23 24 25 26 27 28 1 2 3 4 5 6 7	March
June	1 2 3 4 5 6 7 8 9 10 11 12 13 14 15 16 17 18 19 20 21 22 23 24 25 26 27 28 29 30	June
March	8 9 10 11 12 13 14 15 16 17 18 19 20 21 22 23 24 25 26 27 28 29 30 31 1 2 3 4 5 6	April
July	1 2 3 4 5 6 7 8 9 10 11 12 13 14 15 16 17 18 19 20 21 22 23 24 25 26 27 28 29 30 31	July
April	7 8 9 10 11 12 13 14 15 16 17 18 19 20 21 22 23 24 25 26 27 28 29 30 1 2 3 4 5 6 7	May
August	1 2 3 4 5 6 7 8 9 10 11 12 13 14 15 16 17 18 19 20 21 22 23 24 25 26 27 28 29 30 31	August
May	8 9 10 11 12 13 14 15 16 17 18 19 20 21 22 23 24 25 26 27 28 29 30 31 1 2 3 4 5 6 7	June
September	1 2 3 4 5 6 7 8 9 10 11 12 13 14 15 16 17 18 19 20 21 22 23 24 25 26 27 28 29 30	September
June	8 9 10 11 12 13 14 15 16 17 18 19 20 21 22 23 24 25 26 27 28 29 30 1 2 3 4 5 6 7	July
October	1 2 3 4 5 6 7 8 9 10 11 12 13 14 15 16 17 18 19 20 21 22 23 24 25 26 27 28 29 30 31	October
July	8 9 10 11 12 13 14 15 16 17 18 19 20 21 22 23 24 25 26 27 28 29 30 31 1 2 3 4 5 6 7	August
November	1 2 3 4 5 6 7 8 9 10 11 12 13 14 15 16 17 18 19 20 21 22 23 24 25 26 27 28 29 30	November
August	8 9 10 11 12 13 14 15 16 17 18 19 20 21 22 23 24 25 26 27 28 29 30 31 1 2 3 4 5 6	September
December	1 2 3 4 5 6 7 8 9 10 11 12 13 14 15 16 17 18 19 20 21 22 23 24 25 26 27 28 29 30 31	December
September	7 8 9 10 11 12 13 14 15 16 17 18 19 20 21 22 23 24 25 26 27 28 29 30 1 2 3 4 5 6 7	October

Find the first day of your last period on the pink band. The date on the lighter tint below is your estimated date of delivery (EDD).

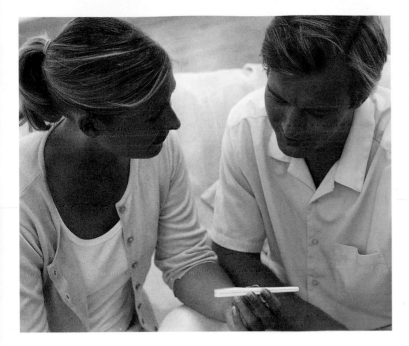

The moment you and your partner know that you are definitely pregnant can be very special for you both. A home test can confirm a pregnancy on the day that your period is due.

usually shown as a coloured line in the window of the testing strip. The colour may be quite faint, particularly if you are doing the test early on. However, this still counts as a positive result.

The amount of HCG in a woman's body doubles every two or three days during the first six weeks of pregnancy. If a test is negative but your period still does not start, it is worth repeating the test in another two or three days. If the second result is also negative, you are probably not pregnant. See your family doctor for confirmation if you are still unsure.

For optimum results, it can be helpful to do a pregnancy test early in the morning, when HCG is present in its greatest concentrations. However, most modern tests are very sensitive, and they should give an accurate reading at any time of day. You can do the test on the day that your period is due.

How reliable are pregnancy tests?

Pregnancy tests are extremely reliable – if you get a positive result you are almost certainly pregnant. However sometimes women do the test wrongly or read the result incorrectly. Very occasionally the test fails to work properly or there is not enough HCG to show a positive result. If you are unsure about a result, you can ask your doctor to do a test for you: you will need to provide a urine sample while you are at the surgery.

Finding out that you are not pregnant can be very disappointing. It is important for you and your partner to take some time to recover from the disappointment and to talk about how you both feel.

A POSITIVE RESULT

If the result of your test is positive, make an appointment to see your doctor two or three weeks later – when you are about eight weeks pregnant. If you are on any medication, see your doctor sooner – the medication may need to be adjusted to ensure that it does not interfere with the healthy development of your baby.

What a doctor will do

Your doctor will confirm the pregnancy by doing another pregnancy test. He or she will check that you are taking folic acid and will also ask you about your general health.

You may be offered an ultrasound scan to date the pregnancy if you are not sure when your last period started. A scan through the abdominal wall will show the baby's heartbeat at seven weeks from the last period, so long as you are not overweight. If you are overweight or if the pregnancy is less than seven weeks, a scan through the vagina may be recommended. A vaginal scan can feel slightly uncomfortable, but it does not increase the risk of miscarriage nor does it cause any harm to the baby.

If you have symptoms such as bleeding or pelvic discomfort, a vaginal scan may be done to check that the pregnancy has not established itself outside the uterus (an ectopic pregnancy). This is important because an ectopic pregnancy can be life-threatening if left untreated.

Common Qs and As

Q: After several months of trying to get pregnant, I am now starting to think about nothing else. I wait for my fertile period, both of us have cut down on alcohol to a couple of glasses of wine a week, I make sure that neither of us is tired out before my fertile period... and then within two or three weeks, I get yet another period. I am starting to feel depressed about this and am beginning to believe that we will never have a family. What can we do?

A: First and foremost, try to relax, by any means that appeals to you. Make sure that you get enough exercise, and join a yoga or relaxation class. Make sure that both you and your partner are sleeping well: invest in a better bed if necessary.

Some couples do not become pregnant for two or more years, even though there is nothing wrong with either partner. Most gynaecologists know of hundreds of cases in which conception is delayed and then, for no obvious reason, the problem resolves and the woman becomes pregnant.

The single most important thing for couples in this situation to remember is that they should never give up hope. What is known as unexplained infertility can just as easily, in time, give way to unexplained fertility. In the meantime, it is important to recognize the effect of repeated monthly disappointments on one's partner and the impact of delayed conception on you in respect of your other relationships and your family, as well as on how you manage at work.

Beware of damaging your relationship with your life partner for the sake of a need that may develop into an obsession with fertility and having children at some time in the future. If you are not pregnant after one year of trying, consult your family doctor with a view to a specialist referral.

Q: We have been trying for a baby now for four months and I am becoming increasingly worried and upset. Should we visit our family doctor, or is it too soon?

A: One in six couples experience delays and difficulties in conception. This is nothing unusual. It may take a year or more for you to become pregnant. See your doctor now if you prefer to do so, but you could probably afford to wait for a few months. It may well be that you find yourself pregnant before you see him or her.

Q: We have been trying for a baby for over one year now. I want to consult our family doctor but my partner is unwilling to do so. What can I do? Do you think this is a sign that he is less committed to the idea of starting a family than I am?

A: The fact that you are not yet pregnant may be worrying him. He may be feeling inadequate and disappointed. Talk to him and try to find out why he is so unwilling. He may fear that the issue lies with him, rather than you. Tell him that male fertility problems account for only one-third of cases – even a low sperm count, if that is what it turns out to be, does not make pregnancy impossible. Explain that there may be a relatively simple problem, such as a cyst or a blocked tube. Once he knows some of the facts, he may be more willing to seek help.

It might be helpful to drop the subject and concentrate on reassuring your partner and showing him that you love him for a month or so. However, you would be wise to see your doctor before too much more time passes. If your partner is still unwilling, make an appointment for yourself.

Q : I am getting very worried that there is a problem with me as my wife and I have been trying to get pregnant for nearly a year now, with no success. I'm concerned that I may be doing something wrong. I eat well and have given up smoking, but I have had a very pressured time at work over the last year and am probably drinking more than I should. I also had some kidney problems a year or so ago.

A : There are many reasons why conception does not happen straight away, but it may well be that your sperm count is low as a combined result of tiredness and alcohol. Alcohol has been shown to contribute to lower sperm counts, and fatigue can also do this, at least partly because it is probably making you less inclined to make love. However, kidney disease is another possible factor, as it can also lower sperm production, so do consult your family doctor about this.

Q : Both of my aunts had fibroids and this affected their ability to get pregnant. How do you know if you have them?

A : The problem with fibroids (non-cancerous growths) is that you don't know they are there. The only symptoms tend to be heavy menstrual bleeding, including flooding, very long-lasting periods, and feelings of exhaustion or depression. If you suffer any of these symptoms, you should see your family doctor without delay for diagnosis and treatment.

Q : My partner and I are discussing the possibility of assisted conception treatment. We are concerned that the success rates are so low, and are not sure whether it is worth going ahead or not.

A : Assisted conception treatments do have a low success rate, and most couples have to undergo several cycles of treatment before conceiving. There are obviously no guarantees of success here.

Some couples decide that assisted conception is not for them, and find other ways of coming to terms with their infertility. Only you can decide whether or not you want to go ahead. You should be offered counselling so that you can explore the issues fully – ask your specialist for a referral.

Q : I am not sure how keen my partner is to start a family, although he has agreed that we should and we have been trying for a while. Almost like clockwork, as soon as my fertile period is about to start, we have a row and do not make love for a few days. Then – once I am no longer fertile – we make it up. I have been thinking that it is simply coincidence, but now I am not sure. How can I stop this happening?

A : Consider whether your anxiety about conceiving is playing a part in this situation. It could be that you feel so tense when approaching your fertile period that a disagreement becomes inevitable. Alternatively, it could be that your partner does have real doubts about having a family.

The only way through this is to talk about the issue. Choose a time when you are both calm, and make sure that you listen to what he has to say. You may find it helpful to seek relationship counselling (via your family doctor or specialist organizations) to explore the issues further.

CHAPTER FIVE
Natural therapies

❝ Natural therapies can provide a really positive cornerstone to your preconception programme. **❞**

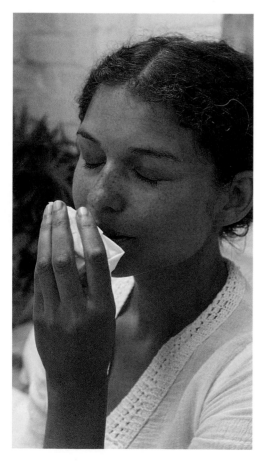

The aim of this chapter is to give in-depth background to, and additional information on, the natural therapies mentioned in the main body of the book. To give you the full picture, and because you may already have conceived, there is information here both for those at the hopeful pre-conception stage and for women who are pregnant.

The many natural therapies that are now available can provide a really positive cornerstone to your preconception care programme. While there is a wide range of opinion on whether therapies such as yoga or herbalism can actually physically promote conception in any way, few would deny that such therapies can provide enormous support throughout the emotional highs and lows experienced by most people trying for a baby. As for the physical aspect, anything that promotes a healthier body will help to ease the path to a better pregnancy and an easier birth and prepare both parents for the demands of looking after a baby.

The benefits of aromatherapy can be enjoyed in many different ways, from adding oils to your bath to sniffing a few drops on a handkerchief.

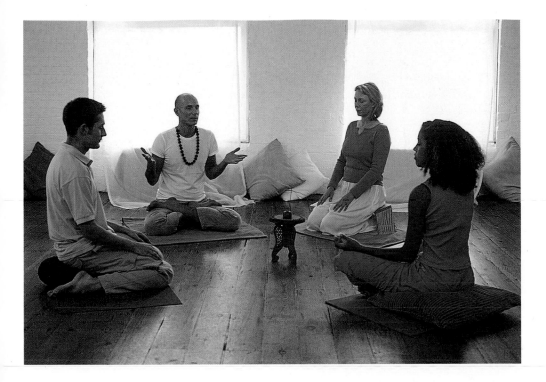

It cannot be stated enough that you must choose only qualified practitioners and ideally seek the advice of your doctor before embarking on any treatment or form of exercise. Remember when you are trying for a baby that you could already be pregnant and the early stages of pregnancy can be vulnerable ones. Don't be terrified of any therapy as soon as you start to try for a baby, but do take sensible precautions. For example, Pilates is a dynamic form of exercise where pregnant women should not do all of the same exercises as others. So if you are actively trying to conceive, let your instructor know before you start classes. Be careful, but do enjoy yourself and pick a therapy that suits you – that way you will be sure to stick with it.

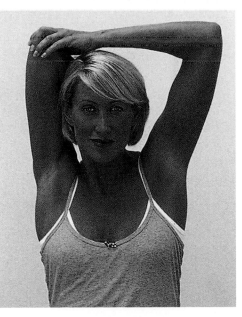

Top: Meditation can bring much-needed mental stillness at this challenging time. You may want to enjoy it as a couple by joining a group class.

Regular yoga and simple stretching exercises help to improve breathing technique and pelvic flexibility as well as calming the mind and emotions.

Herbalism

Many plants have therapeutic properties, which can be used to improve health and treat illness. Researchers are currently substantiating many of the claims made for herbal remedies. For the mother-to-be, herbs can offer support in all kinds of ways, from calming anxiety to alleviating morning sickness.

Many modern medicines are derived from plants. Science has made it possible to isolate the active ingredients or recreate entirely synthetic versions, so pharmaceutical drugs are now far removed from their natural origins. By contrast, herbal remedies use parts of the whole plant – roots, seeds, petals or leaves. Herbalists say that the subtle interaction of all the herb's ingredients promotes healing in a holistic (whole body) way rather than merely attacking a single symptom or disease as many laboratory-produced drugs do.

HERBAL MEDICINE AND PREGNANCY

Women have long used herbal remedies to alleviate the discomforts of pregnancy, prepare the body for childbirth, and aid recovery afterwards. Herbalists say that remedies can also be used to enhance fertility.

Herbal medicines are usually gentler than chemical ones, but this is not always the case. It is important to bear in mind that herbal remedies can have powerful effects. This is very important during pregnancy, when many herbs should not be used. It is not a good idea to self-prescribe herbal remedies, particularly if you are trying to conceive or are pregnant. See a qualified medical herbalist for advice.

SEEING A HERBALIST

When you see a herbalist, a medical history will be taken and you will be given a physical examination. You should tell your practitioner about any drugs you are taking since they may interact badly with natural remedies; for the same reason, tell your doctor about any remedies you are given. A medical herbalist will advise you on your diet and lifestyle

SAFETY REMINDERS
- Never take a herbal remedy unless you are sure that it is safe. Consult a qualified herbalist for advice.
- Tell your doctor or midwife about any remedies you are taking.
- Do not exceed the recommended dosage.
- Contact your practitioner or doctor immediately if you suffer any ill effects.

as well as prescribing remedies for your individual needs. You will usually have at least one follow-up appointment; often several sessions will be necessary.

SELF-HELP HERBAL REMEDIES

One of the areas where herbs can be used during pre-conception is in helping to boost immunity. Many people believe that a healthy immune system promotes your chances of conceiving. In any case, immunity lowers naturally during early pregnancy, so getting it into good shape is advisable for the health of any mother-to-be and her baby. Echinacea, garlic and lemon balm are good choices, and all of these are safe to continue taking once pregnant. Drink no more than three cups of herbal tea a day. Other ways of taking herbs include pills, capsules, drops, ointments, compresses and poultices.

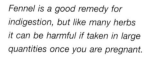

Fennel is a good remedy for indigestion, but like many herbs it can be harmful if taken in large quantities once you are pregnant.

HERBS TO AVOID PRE- AND POST-CONCEPTION

- angelica
- barberry
- black cohosh
- bloodroot
- buckthorn
- celery
- cinchona
- cinnamon
- cottonroot
- feverfew
- golden seal
- greater celandine
- juniper
- liferoot
- male fern
- mandrake
- mistletoe
- mugwort
- nutmeg
- pennyroyal
- poke root
- rhubarb
- rosemary
- rue
- saffron
- sage
- southernwood
- tansy
- thuja
- thyme
- wormwood

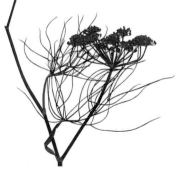

Homeopathy

This gentle therapy can help with many of the physical symptoms and difficult emotions experienced while trying to conceive and during pregnancy. The remedies are derived from natural substances, and aim to stimulate the body's capacity for healing and restore well-being.

Homeopathy is based on the idea that 'like cures like': so a substance that causes illness can also be used to cure it. The remedies have been so diluted that only the merest trace of the active ingredient remains. In this state, they are far too weak to cause harm, but homeopaths believe that the minute dose can promote self-healing and cure the very symptoms that it might cause if taken in large amounts. Some doctors are sceptical about homeopathic remedies, but others accept that they can have good results. Some have trained in this therapy and offer it to patients as an adjunct to orthodox medical care.

Homeopathic remedies are considered very safe pre- and post-conception. They can help to relieve many ailments, from anxiety to morning sickness, and to speed recovery after birth. Self-help remedies are available from many pharmacies, but it can be difficult to choose exactly the right one for you. For this reason, it is much better to consult a homeopath.

SEEING A HOMEOPATH

A homeopath will take a full personal and medical history during the first session, which can last two hours. People are often surprised by the number and type of questions they are asked. However, the homeopath needs to build up a picture of your habits and preferences as well as your mental, physical and emotional make-up. This information enables him or her to assess your 'constitutional type'.

Homeopaths consider both the patient's constitution and symptoms when choosing from the 2,000 remedies at their disposal. You will be given instructions on how to take the remedies, and may also be given advice about your diet and lifestyle. A follow-up appointment is usually arranged; often several sessions are necessary.

EFFECTIVE HOMEOPATHY

- See a homeopath who is experienced in treating pregnant women; tell him or her if you are pregnant or are trying to conceive.
- Follow the homeopath's instructions when taking the remedy: for example, avoid drinking or eating for 15 minutes after taking a remedy.
- Contact your homeopath if your symptoms worsen (this may be part of the healing process).
- Tell your doctor about any remedies you take, and report any unusual symptoms.

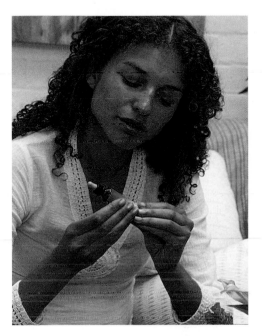

Flower remedies are a useful 'instant cure', and can be used to help resolve uncomfortable emotions, such as self-doubt, anxiety or low spirits.

BACH FLOWER REMEDIES

The Bach Flower Remedies are homeopathic remedies preserved in grape alcohol. Plant-based, they are designed to help with negative feelings or states of mind. The most popular is Rescue Remedy, which is used for panic, tearfulness or shock. The remedies are available from health-food shops and pharmacies, and are usually self-prescribed.

To take a flower remedy, place a few drops in a glass of water and sip. Repeat several times a day if you are struggling with a recurring emotion. Flower remedies are preserved in alcohol, but you take only a tiny amount so they are safe for use in pregnancy. See your doctor if you are at all unsure about whether or not you should use them.

Aromatherapy

Aromatherapists use aromatic oils extracted from herbs and flowers to promote well-being. Aromatherapy oils smell wonderful and are very pleasurable to use. They can be a gentle and effective way of boosting general health and treating minor ailments and are excellent for promoting relaxation.

We do not know exactly how essential oils work, but it is thought that the scents trigger a reaction in smell receptors in the nostrils, which send messages to the brain. When the oils are used in massage, they also penetrate the skin and have a direct effect on the nerve endings here.

Some of the oils have proven medicinal qualities: tea tree, for example, is an antiseptic, antifungal and antibacterial agent, while chamomile has antispasmodic and antidepressant properties. Lavender is one of the most versatile oils: it helps with stress, insomnia, migraine and headaches, and it can also promote healing after a burn.

BENEFITS OF AROMATHERAPY

Most people find that aromatherapy's main benefit is relaxation – very helpful while trying to conceive. It can also help to induce general feelings of well-being, reduce fatigue and relieve backache. Once you are pregnant, essential oils can be used to help the circulation, and so reduce the likelihood of varicose veins and haemorrhoids.

Never use an oil unless you have checked that it is safe for those trying to conceive or already pregnant – some stimulate the uterus, causing miscarriage, and it may be safest to avoid using essential oils entirely in the early weeks.

SEEING AN AROMATHERAPIST

Aromatherapists are usually trained masseurs. During the first session, a practitioner will ask you about your medical history and any current health problems. You should say if

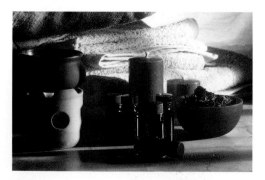

One of the gentlest ways to use essential oils is to heat them in a vaporizer. Their scent will fill a room and have an uplifting or relaxing effect upon everyone in it.

you are trying to conceive, or are already pregnant, and should ideally see an aromatherapist who regularly works with conceiving or pregnant women. The therapist will choose up to five oils, blended in a carrier such as almond oil. You will be asked to undress and lie on a couch and the therapist will massage the oils into your skin. You should be given a few minutes to rest at the end of the session.

SELF-HELP AROMATHERAPY

The following methods can be used for self-help at home.

BATHS

Aromatherapy baths are very relaxing. A warm bath with a soothing oil such as Roman chamomile can promote restful sleep. Mix four to six drops of essential oil with a carrier oil or whole milk, then add to a full bath (not to running water). Lie back in the bath and breathe deeply, for 10–15 minutes.

MASSAGE

Self-massage is a great way of applying oils. An essential oil should always be well-diluted in a vegetable oil, such as jojoba, sesame or almond: use a dilution of one drop per 5ml/1 tsp base oil (or per 10ml/2 tsp if you are pregnant).

INHALATION

The simplest method is to put two drops of essential oil on to a tissue, and inhale. Slip a tissue with Roman chamomile on it under your pillowcase to encourage sleep. For a steam inhalation, put five drops of essential oil into a bowl of hot water. Cover your head and the bowl with a towel, and breathe (eyes closed).

Massage
Touch has been used to enhance health for thousands of years and is a powerful way of giving comfort and relieving pain: we instinctively hug a friend in distress or rub an aching limb. This leading touch therapy can be especially useful in eliminating toxins and so can help to get the body in top shape for conception.

The term 'massage' covers many different therapies. On the one hand, there is purely physical Western massage, which works on the muscles. On the other, there are forms of Eastern pressure massage, which seek to enhance energy flow along invisible pathways in the body. These include shiatsu and acupressure. Massage techniques also form an important element of therapies such as osteopathy, aromatherapy and reflexology.

SWEDISH MASSAGE
In the West, most therapists practise Swedish massage. This system was devised by a Swedish gymnast, Per Henrik Ling, in the late 18th century. The techniques include:
- **Stroking** (effleurage) to relax. Firmer strokes are used to stimulate the circulation and release muscular tension.
- **Kneading** (petrissage) which soothes tense muscles and increases blood flow to particular areas. It can be used to relax deep muscles, such as those of the shoulders.
- **Friction** in which small, circular movements are made with the pads of the thumbs. It is used to break down areas of muscular spasm.
- **Percussion** in which fast, rhythmic movements are performed with the sides of the hands on fleshy parts of the body. It should be avoided during pregnancy.

RECEIVING A MASSAGE
To receive a Swedish massage, you'll be asked to undress and lie on a special couch. However, you can keep your underwear on if you wish. Towels will be placed over any areas of your body not being massaged. The therapist will usually massage your whole body, but may spend longer on some areas and leave out others. He or she will use oil or cream to prevent any dragging of the skin. The session typically lasts an hour, and you will usually be left to relax for a few minutes at the end.

Benefits of Swedish massage
There has been a great deal of research into massage, and most doctors accept that it promotes general good health. Having a massage is a good habit to acquire: its relaxing effects help many people to deal with the anxiety that often accompanies trying to conceive, then those who become pregnant can use it to ease backache, joint pain, blood pressure and digestive problems, headaches and insomnia. Stroking the lower back during labour may soothe pain.

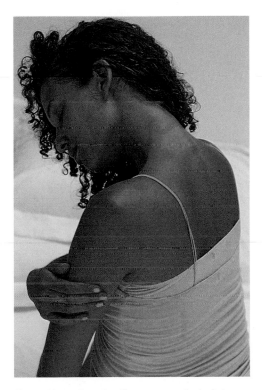

Pleasurable touch on the skin encourages the body to release endorphins, natural pain-killing chemicals. These help to induce feelings of well-being and can ease all kinds of pain and discomfort.

Effective massage before and during pregnancy
Check with your doctor or midwife before having massage in pregnancy. Seek out a therapist who is experienced in treating pregnant women.
- Tell the therapist that you are trying to conceive/pregnant.
- You should not have deep pressure on the abdomen or lower back if there is a chance that you are pregnant.
- Varicose veins, bruises or lumps must not be massaged.
- Do not have a massage if you have an infection or fever or if you feel unwell.
- Drink plenty of water and avoid strenuous activity afterwards. If possible, rest.

Yoga
Doctors and midwives now commonly recommend yoga to pregnant women. This ancient form of exercise is known to foster general good health and improve posture and flexibility. It can also help to prevent or relieve common ailments such as backache, constipation and headaches.

Yoga is proven to help people relax, which makes it highly beneficial for women who are trying to conceive or who are already pregnant. Regular practice can help to strengthen the body and loosen up the pelvis in preparation for the birth; it can also aid recovery afterwards.

Most yoga practised by Westerners is a form of hatha yoga. This means that it involves physical postures (asanas) as well as breath-control techniques, meditation and relaxation exercises. Certain poses, such as spinal twists and headstands, should be avoided by those who might be or are pregnant. Seek out classes taught by someone with knowledge of pregnancy issues – there are now classes for promoting conception as well as for pregnancy. If you are pregnant and want to take up yoga for the first time, it is best to wait until you are past the 12-week mark before starting classes. If you already practise a well-established yoga routine, it should be safe to continue in the first trimester, but work gently and avoid unsuitable postures.

YOGA PRACTICE

In yoga, everyone works to his or her own capacity. It is important that you do not push yourself any further than you are naturally able to go. With practice, your body will become stronger and more flexible. In many yoga classes, equipment is available to help you work with the postures.

Yoga classes vary widely, depending on the form being taught and the teacher's training and interest. They usually last 1–1½ hours. Generally, you will start with easy postures,

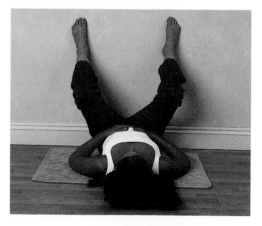

CHOOSING A YOGA TEACHER
Anyone can teach yoga, and standards do vary. Before committing to a class, ask your yoga teacher about his or her experience and training – reputable teachers should be happy to discuss this. Your teacher should also be insured. Pregnant women should only attend 'yoga for pregnancy' classes.

which warm up the body, and then move on to more advanced ones. Usually, sitting, standing, reclining and some inversions (adapted if you are pregnant) are covered.

The teacher will demonstrate each posture, then explain the series of movements needed to get into it, plus simplified versions of the postures where necessary. You may be given individual attention in order to improve your alignment. All postures should be done on a non-slip mat.

The class will end with simple breathing exercises and relaxation. It is vital that you complete the relaxation since it gives the body a chance to cool down. It also helps to calm the mind. Yoga is most effective if you do it regularly. Your teacher will advise you on which postures to do at home.

GETTING THE MOST FROM YOGA

- Always tell your yoga teacher that you are, or may be, pregnant. Mention any health problems that you have.
- Do not eat or drink a large amount of water for an hour before the class; avoid eating a large meal in the three hours beforehand.
- Wear loose, comfortable clothing. Do the poses in bare feet, but put socks on for the relaxation if you wish.
- If you are practising at home, make sure that any postures you do are suitable for you personally.
- Never strain or over-extend your body.
- Breathe freely: do not hold your breath when getting into or out of a posture.
- If you feel faint or uncomfortable, stop and rest on your left side for a few minutes.
- Always end a yoga session with at least ten minutes of relaxation time.

This version of a shoulder-stand helps blood to drain from the legs. It is suitable for pregnancy and may help to prevent varicose veins if done daily.

Meditation

This is a form of mental exercise that can lead to greater inner harmony and awareness, making it the ideal way to relax and deal with the stresses of conception and pregnancy. It developed as a spiritual practice, but you do not have to subscribe to any particular philosophy to enjoy its benefits.

Many doctors believe that relaxation is an important part of general healthcare, and recommend meditation to their patients. Research has shown that regular meditation can reverse the effects of stress and help to alleviate ailments such as insomnia and digestive problems.

Meditation can soothe the emotions and help people to gain a wider perspective. Spending a few minutes each day in quiet contemplation can help women to cope with the disappointments that can be part of trying to conceive, as well as the challenges of pregnancy and new motherhood.

PRACTISING MEDITATION

Meditation practices vary, but they can often involve concentrating on a single object. The simplest way of practising meditation is probably to focus on your own breathing. You can also choose to focus on a physical object such as a flower or a candle flame, or on a sound that you repeat over and over again (known as a mantra). These concentration practices help to still the mind and have a relaxing effect on the body.

VISUALIZATION

This is a form of meditation that involves picturing an object, a happy event or a relaxing, beautiful scene in your mind's eye. It is a recognized technique for self-help and is much used by sportsmen with an athletic goal or achievement in mind.

Visualization can be used to promote well-being; in pregnancy, it may be helpful for easing anxiety and promoting bonding. For example, imagine a baby being successfully conceived inside you and growing healthily, or visualize healing pink or golden light surrounding you and your child.

LEARNING MEDITATION

You can learn basic meditative techniques from a book or tape. Most people find that it is much easier to learn and to concentrate when they are in a group. An experienced teacher will be able to answer any questions that you have. Classes vary widely and it is important that you choose one you feel comfortable with – talk to the teacher beforehand.

Meditation is a gentle technique that can ease anxiety and stress-related symptoms. Many women find it a helpful way of preparing for conception, pregnancy and birth.

SAFETY POINT

Check with your doctor before starting meditation if you have suffered from any form of psychiatric illness in the past. Sometimes meditation can bring up disturbing thoughts and images.

HYPNOTHERAPY

This field has some general links with meditation practices. Hypnotherapists work by inducing a relaxed, trance-like state in their clients – a state in which clients are highly receptive to any suggestions, including suggestions for self-healing and relaxation. This can be particularly helpful in dealing with the hopes and fears surrounding conception, pregnancy and childbirth, for the partner as well as the mother-to-be.

There has been considerable research into hypnotherapy, and many doctors believe that it can be helpful. However, they stress it should be used as an adjunct to medical treatment, not as a substitute.

Choose a serious, qualified practitioner you trust, and check that he or she belongs to a reputable professional association. You should not have hypnosis if you suffer from epilepsy or if you have suffered severe depression in the past.

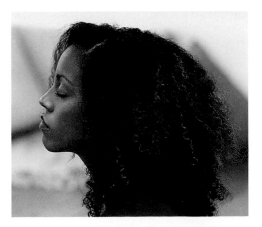

Acupuncture

Practised for centuries in China as a means of promoting good health and treating illness, acupuncture is now widely available in the West, and most doctors accept that it has positive effects. Acupuncture can help with fertility problems and with many pregnancy-related disorders.

Acupuncture is based on the idea that chi (energy) flows along invisible pathways – known as meridians – in the body. When this energy flows freely, good health and well-being are maintained. Illness and emotional upset are said to be a result of blockages or imbalances in the circulation of this energy.

In acupuncture, fine needles are inserted into certain points on the meridians to correct imbalances and improve the flow of chi. Acupuncture is usually practised holistically, so its ultimate aim is to bring the body back to its natural state of equilibrium. However, it can be used to treat specific complaints, such as back pain and digestion problems.

HOW CAN IT HELP?

Acupuncture may ease fertility problems and can relieve many pregnancy-related ailments, including morning sickness, constipation and poor circulation. It may also help with recurrent miscarriage. It is important that you tell your practitioner that you are trying to conceive or are pregnant, as some points should not be stimulated in these cases. For this reason, it is best to choose a qualified practitioner who is experienced in working with pregnant women.

SEEING AN ACUPUNCTURIST

On your first visit, a full medical and personal history will be taken: your practitioner will ask you many questions about, for example, your appetite, bowel movements, sleep and energy levels. Your pulses will be taken and your tongue will be checked. The practitioner will also observe other details, such as the sound of your voice and the colour of your skin.

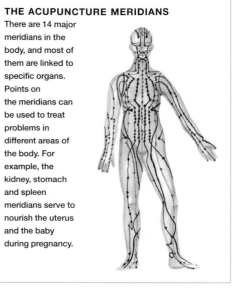

THE ACUPUNCTURE MERIDIANS
There are 14 major meridians in the body, and most of them are linked to specific organs. Points on the meridians can be used to treat problems in different areas of the body. For example, the kidney, stomach and spleen meridians serve to nourish the uterus and the baby during pregnancy.

You lie on a massage couch to receive treatment. The acupuncturist will insert needles into different points on your body – this is swift and painless. Sometimes, the needles will be left in place for several minutes.

Most people have weekly or fortnightly sessions to start with, but you may need only occasional sessions once treatment has been established.

OTHER ACUPUNCTURE TECHNIQUES

Finger pressure can be used instead of needles to stimulate acupoints. Acupressure is less invasive than needling, and it can be used for self-help. Some acupuncturists can advise you and your partner on which points to stimulate during labour.

Another technique is moxibustion, where the herb moxa (mugwort) is burned on energy points. This can exert a profoundly soothing effect.

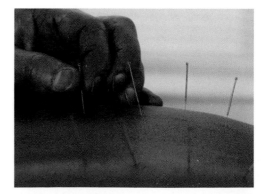

You may feel a slight tingling when an acupuncture needle is inserted, but it should not hurt.

Reflexology

Reflexologists believe that every body part is linked by an energy pathway to a specific point on the foot, and that finger pressure on the feet can detect and treat health problems. Energy levels and immunity can often be boosted with reflexology, so helping to prepare the body for pregnancy.

Reflexology is good for promoting general well-being and relaxation. It can also help alleviate complaints such as back pain, digestive problems and constipation. Some midwives use the techniques to promote regular contractions and for pain relief during labour. One study found that reflexology could reduce a woman's need for pain relief, and cut the length of labour by as much as half.

Many women (and their male partners) enjoy reflexology as a path to well-being prior to conception and also to de-stress and relieve other symptoms during pregnancy. However, ideally reflexology should not be used during the first 12 weeks of pregnancy without close professional supervision. Some areas – the heels, Achilles tendons and ankles – should not be worked on at any stage because this can induce contractions. It is vital to see a practitioner who understands the needs of pregnant women.

SEEING A REFLEXOLOGIST

On your first visit, your practitioner will ask about your medical history, diet, lifestyle and any other therapies you are receiving. You will take off your footwear and sit on a chair or couch. The reflexologist will massage your feet to relax them. After this, every area of your foot will be pressed and massaged in turn. Some areas may feel very

sensitive – this is said to be a sign of imbalance. Tender points will receive extra massage in order to stimulate energy flow to the corresponding area of the body. This can sometimes be painful, but tenderness should ease as the massage continues. Your reflexologist may show you techniques to practise at home. The hands also contain a 'map' of the body, and these are often recommended for self-help as they are easier to treat than the feet.

Like most complementary therapists, reflexologists seek to help the body to heal itself. Regular sessions are often recommended in order to maintain well-being.

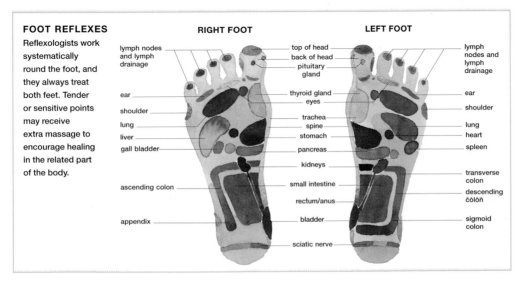

FOOT REFLEXES
Reflexologists work systematically round the foot, and they always treat both feet. Tender or sensitive points may receive extra massage to encourage healing in the related part of the body.

RIGHT FOOT — LEFT FOOT

lymph nodes and lymph drainage
ear
shoulder
lung
liver
gall bladder
ascending colon
appendix

top of head
back of head
pituitary gland
thyroid gland
eyes
trachea
spine
stomach
pancreas
kidneys
small intestine
rectum/anus
bladder
sciatic nerve

lymph nodes and lymph drainage
ear
shoulder
lung
heart
spleen
transverse colon
descending colon
sigmoid colon

Shiatsu

The term shiatsu is Japanese for 'finger pressure'. Practitioners work to stimulate pressure points associated with the vital organs, in order to encourage a good flow of chi (energy) around the body and promote better health. Uses for mothers-to-be include the major issue of maintaining a healthy blood pressure.

Many Japanese people undergo regular shiatsu treatment, sometimes as often as once a week. They believe that it can help to prevent illness as well as detect and treat any symptoms early on. Shiatsu is a holistic system of healing, meaning that the whole person – mind, body and spirit – is treated at once. However, it can also be used to treat problems such as back pain, digestive problems, insomnia, depression, migraine and toothache, and to help strengthen the immune system.

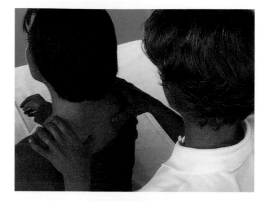

If you think that you might already be pregnant, remember that shiatsu should generally be kept simple and non-specific during the first three months of pregnancy, when the baby's organ systems are developing. To be safe, you should see a practitioner who specializes in working with pregnant women. Shiatsu can help keep your body in the best possible shape for conception and, if you like it, you may want to consider its future use during pregnancy and for natural pain-relief during labour.

SEEING A PRACTITIONER

At the first consultation, a shiatsu practitioner should take a detailed medical and lifestyle history from you. He or she will take your pulses: there are six at each wrist, each associated with a vital organ. He or she may also feel your abdomen, which can give clues to problems elsewhere. The sound of your voice, your appearance and posture will also be observed.

To receive treatment, you lie on a mat on the floor, fully clothed. The practitioner then applies pressure to points all over your body using various different parts of his or her hands: the bulb of the thumb, the fingertips, or the palm or heel of the hand. An elbow may also be used or perhaps a forearm or a knee. The practitioner may perform gentle stretching or rocking movements.

How hard the therapist applies pressure depends on many things, including the part of the body being treated, how you react and whether you require a tonic or a sedating effect. Pressure is applied for a few seconds at a time and is repeated several times at each spot.

You can learn how to apply finger pressure at home after learning the techniques from a trained shiatsu practitioner.

Shiatsu practitioners often use finger pressure (top) to activate an energy point, but they also use the whole hand, the forearm (right), the elbows or the feet.

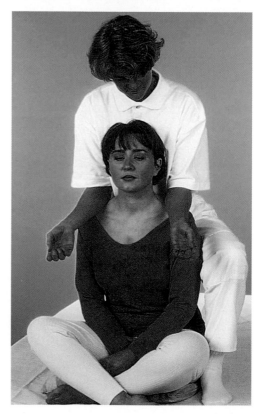

Osteopathy

Osteopaths believe that good health depends on the proper functioning of our muscles and joints. They use manipulation and massage to correct imbalances caused by injury, poor posture and stress. Their approach can be especially helpful in easing digestive problems and headaches.

Most people see an osteopath because of backache, but the therapy can also help with other physical problems, such as headaches, digestive disorders and breathing difficulties. Osteopathy is safe in pregnancy, but you should be sure to choose a qualified practitioner with experience in treating pregnant women: osteopathic techniques can be dangerous if performed by an untrained practitioner.

You should always tell your osteopath if you are trying to conceive or are already pregnant, and let your doctor know that you are having treatment. Some doctors will be able to recommend an osteopath to you.

WHAT TO EXPECT

An osteopath will take a full medical and lifestyle history on your first visit, and he or she will also give you a physical examination. People are usually asked to undress to their underwear so that the osteopath can observe the body's framework.

The practitioner will use gentle touch – palpation – to detect any areas of weakness or strain in your body. You may be asked to perform simple exercises while standing, sitting and lying on a couch so that your osteopath can check your posture, muscle tone and breathing technique. Sometimes other medical tests – such as blood tests – will be carried out to help with diagnosis.

CRANIAL OSTEOPATHY

Some osteopaths practise cranial osteopathy. This gentle technique focuses on the delicate manipulation of the bones of the skull in order to improve the circulation of blood and fluid in the head. It is said to help many of the same conditions as conventional osteopathy, and it is often used to help babies who are suffering from sleeplessness, colic or birth trauma.

In cranial-sacral therapy, subtle pressure is applied to the head and the base of the spine. Therapists are aiming to regulate the flow of cerebrospinal fluid, which affects the whole nervous system and thus the functioning of the body. Many people find this therapy deeply relaxing, and it can help with insomnia, backache and headaches.

Doctors tend to be more sceptical of these gentle techniques than of conventional osteopathy, but many patients report good results. Some cranial-sacral therapists may not have undergone the rigorous training of an osteopath. Seek treatment only from qualified osteopaths or chiropractors with experience in dealing with pregnant women and babies.

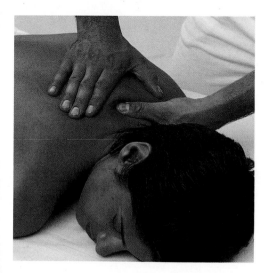

You lie on a massage couch for treatment. The osteopath will then carry out a series of manipulations, which are tailored to your individual needs. The techniques used include massage, limb stretches and sharp thrusts. You may hear a clicking sound as a joint slips back into alignment, but you should not feel any pain.

The first session can last an hour but subsequent treatments are usually 20–30 minutes long. Most people need several sessions, and you may also be given instructions on exercises to do at home.

Pregnant women are often advised to have regular sessions to help them adjust to changes in their posture as the baby grows. This is a good way of preventing and treating lower back pain. Some osteopaths say that regular treatment during pregnancy can help to make the birth easier.

Many people are nervous of the clicking sound that occurs when an osteopath pops a joint back into place. However, this should not be painful. Treatment also includes gentle massage and stretches, which are very relaxing.

Chiropractic

Chiropractors use their hands to work on the spine, believing that a well-aligned spine is vital in maintaining good health because it supports the rest of the body and houses the central nervous system. One major use is to ease back problems in preparation for carrying a growing baby.

Chiropractic is mainly used to help with back and neck problems. Gentle manipulation of the spine is performed to improve posture, and to correct any kinks caused by injury or stress. Regular sessions of chiropractic can help pregnant women to adjust their posture so that they cope better with the strain of carrying a growing baby. It may also alleviate pelvic problems and make childbirth easier.

Chiropractics say that working on the spine can also help seemingly unrelated problems. This is because nerve pathways branch off the spine at different levels and travel to all areas of the body. Distortions in the spine can affect nerve function, and may therefore be the cause of problems elsewhere. Fatigue, indigestion, constipation and headaches may all be helped by chiropractic treatment.

SEEING A CHIROPRACTOR

Your first session will focus mainly on the diagnosis of your problem. A full medical history will be taken and you will also be asked questions about your work, lifestyle and diet, and any exercise that you do.

You will be asked to undress to your underwear so that the chiropractor can observe your closely. If you feel embarrassed, you may be able to wear a gown. The chiropractor will observe your posture as you sit, stand and

THE ORTHODOX VIEW

Chiropractic is widely accepted as a useful technique for many back problems. However, many doctors are sceptical about claims that it can help with problems such as digestive disorders.

OTHER FORMS OF CHIROPRACTIC THERAPY

Practitioners of McTimoney or McTimoney-Corley chiropractic use many of the same techniques as conventional chiropractors, but they tend to work in a more gentle way.

McTimoney chiropractors agree that the distortions in the spine are the principle cause of ill health but they think that all other joints should be treated as well. They examine and work on the whole musculoskeletal system in each treatment session. McTimoney-Corley chiropractic is different again: practitioners manipulate the vertebrae using their fingertips, and they do not practise the more vigorous techniques of chiropractic. They emphasize the importance of self-help exercises.

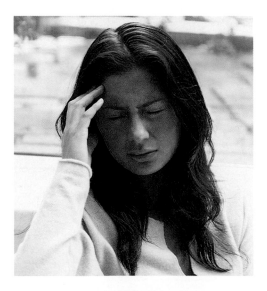

lie down, and you will be asked to perform some simple exercises. The chiropractor may check the mobility of your joints by asking you to perform a few stretches. He or she will then examine your spine to detect any misalignments or areas of stiffness, as well as the source of any pain you may have. Other checks, such as blood pressure or reflex tests, may also be performed.

You will be asked to lie on a massage couch for treatment. The chiropractor will use a variety of techniques to realign the vertebrae: these include gentle stretches, precise thrusts and massage. You may ache or feel rather stiff afterwards, but the treatment should not hurt.

Most people need several sessions of chiropractic, but you may start to see some improvement in your condition after just one treatment.

Chiropractors are able to treat much more than just back problems. For example, regular headaches and bouts of indigestion may also be relieved by releasing built-up tension in the spine.

The Alexander technique

In this therapy, gentle posture-improving exercises show clients how to stand, sit and move. This eases pressure on muscles and joints and is held to relieve all kinds of mental and physical problems, from anxiety about conception to the strain of carrying a heavy 'bump'.

As children, we have naturally good posture. However, as we grow up we tend to develop bad habits: we may slouch or cross our legs when we sit, stand with our weight pushed on to one leg, and twist the back when lifting. Our mental state, too, can affect our posture: when stressed we may lift the shoulders and hold them in a state of tension, for example, and the problem may be compounded by poor sitting technique and by working at a computer.

Eventually, these habits, known as 'patterns of misuse', become ingrained. Poor posture becomes the norm, and we no longer notice when we are placing the body under strain. Over time, poor posture causes damage to our muscles and joints, and our digestive, respiratory and circulatory systems may also be affected.

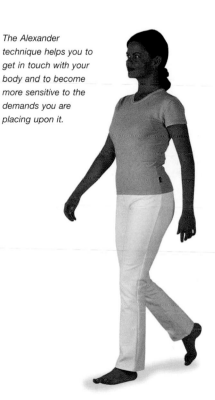

The Alexander technique helps you to get in touch with your body and to become more sensitive to the demands you are placing upon it.

HOW THE ALEXANDER TECHNIQUE WORKS

The Alexander technique is a way of training people to become aware of bad habits, so that they can start to stand and move in a naturally better way. It emphasizes aligning the head with the spine, so that the neck remains free of strain. The technique is best taught on a one-to-one basis. During the first session, you will be asked to adopt various positions and perform simple movements, while the teacher observes how you stand, sit and move.

You will be asked to lie down, and the teacher will make subtle adjustments to your limbs, head, pelvis and so on, so that you can experience good posture for yourself.

During the classes, the teacher will show you how to perform a whole range of everyday tasks in the Alexander way – such as answering the telephone, getting in and out of a chair, writing a letter, answering the phone, carrying a bag, and walking. The lessons will combine gentle manipulations with verbal instructions. The aim is to build your awareness of how to move correctly – called 'thought in action'. Eventually, you will be able to bring this awareness into daily life, and maintain good posture.

Sessions are usually given once or twice a week for several months; thereafter top-up sessions may be needed.

HOW IT HELPS

The Alexander technique is accepted as an effective way of treating many back and neck problems. Practitioners say that posture work can also help people to become more resistant to stress. Other conditions that may be helped by the technique include depression, anxiety, headaches, high blood pressure, infertility, breathing problems, fatigue, arthritis, back pain and digestive disorders.

ONCE YOU ARE PREGNANT

The Alexander technique can help pregnant women adapt to their changing shape as the baby grows. This may prevent the backache that is commonly associated with pregnancy.

It will also help you to prepare for the birth. The Alexander technique teaches women to stay upright during labour – in a squatting position – so that the force of gravity can assist the baby's passage. An Alexander teacher will help you to learn how to cope with contractions without tensing the body. This can make childbirth easier, since tension increases pain.

Pilates
This is an effective form of body conditioning, which also develops mental awareness and an effective breathing technique. Some Pilates exercises are similar to yoga postures, but they are repeated to create a flowing sequence. Like yoga, Pilates is excellent at building strength in and around the spine.

Pilates aims to bring the body back to its natural alignment. The exercises encourage you to work to your maximum capability, without placing undue strain on the body. As a result, regular practice helps to improve your posture and flexibility, as well as toning the muscles. Pilates is particularly good for developing 'core' strength in the lower back and abdomen. It aims to work the mind as well as the body, and many practitioners find it deeply relaxing.

Pilates was originally developed in the First World War as a means of helping injured soldiers regain their mobility. It is still often recommended as a form of rehabilitation. Teachers say that almost anyone can practise Pilates because the exercises involved can be adapted to suit the individual's needs.

Pilates is safe for pregnant women because it uses carefully controlled movements and encourages you to work within your body's limitations. Advocates say that it can help to reduce backache, ease delivery and hasten recovery after the birth. However, it is important that the exercises are done correctly. Seek out a specialist qualified teacher who regularly works with pregnant women.

LEARNING PILATES
There are many books on Pilates, but it is best to learn the exercise from a qualified and experienced instructor. Pilates can be learned on a one-to-one basis or in a small class.

Some exercises are practised on a mat and others are done on specialized apparatus. The teacher demonstrates the exercises, and then guides the students through each series of movements. You should receive individual attention, even in a group class, and be shown how to adapt exercises where necessary. Blocks and supports may be used to help you to do this.

Classes usually last an hour. However, once you have learned the techniques, mat exercises can be done at home. Pilates teachers say that it is important to practise three or four times a week in order to obtain the most benefit from this therapy.

SAFE PILATES
- Do not push your body further than is comfortable: you will build up flexibility and strength with practice.
- If you feel uncomfortable at any point, stop and rest.
- Build up slowly – it will take time for you to increase your flexibility and strength.
- If you are pregnant and new to Pilates, do not start classes until after the first trimester. Try to find special pregnancy classes. Otherwise, go for individual instruction with an experienced teacher.
- Exercises where you lie flat on your back should be safe for the first 30 weeks of pregnancy, but not after.

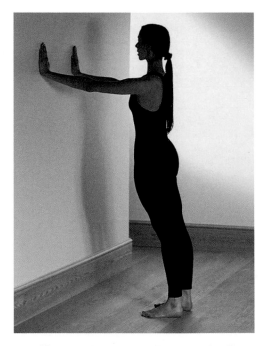

Many Pilates exercises are seemingly easy stretches like this one. When done correctly, they quickly build strength and muscle tone.

CHOOSING A TEACHER
Anyone can call themselves a Pilates teacher – even if they have had just a few days' training. It is important that you check that your teacher has completed a reputable training course and that he or she has been practising Pilates for several years. All Pilates teachers should have insurance.

Glossary

Amniocentesis This is a specialized test that involves taking fluid from the amniotic cavity (amnion). The amnion is the inner sac that surrounds the baby inside the uterus. The cells contained within the fluid can be analysed and also grown in a tissue culture. Together, the results provide information about chromosomal defects, the sex of the baby, inherited disorders, and open neural tube defects.

Amniotic fluid The fluid contained within the amnion. See **Amniocentesis**.

Antenatal This simply means 'before birth' and so relates to the health and care of pregnant women (as in antenatal classes).

AI Process in which the woman is inseminated with her partner's sperm by means of a syringe while she is ovulating. See pages 60–9.

Donor insemination See pages 60–9.

Eclampsia see **pre-eclampsia**.

Ectopic pregnancy This occurs when the fertilized egg implants not in the uterus but elsewhere, in the abdomen or in the Fallopian tubes. Symptoms include bleeding and abdominal pain, sometimes severe, and pain in the shoulder. Immediate hospital admission is required.

Egg donation See pages 60–77.

Embryo The fertilized egg that eventually becomes the developing baby is known as the embryo during the first eight weeks of life. After eight weeks it is known as a fetus, up until birth.

Endorphins The feel-good hormones that are released during exercise (and also during lovemaking) and continue to make us feel good and relieve pain for some time after the exercise itself has stopped.

Fertile period The woman's fertile period lasts for a few days around ovulation. Ovulation itself takes place 14 days before the expected next period. This is not the same as saying that it takes place 14 days after the last period because women's menstrual cycles vary in length very considerably. They can sometimes be as short as 21 days or as long as 38 days rather than the standard 28.

Fetoscopy This procedure involves a microscope camera being inserted into the woman's uterus through the abdomen, in much the same way as occurs in amniocentesis, so that the fetus can be photographed. By sampling tissue like this it may be possible to diagnose several blood and skin diseases that the amniocentesis test cannot. In some centres, certain fetal conditions can be treated before delivery by means of a fetoscopy.

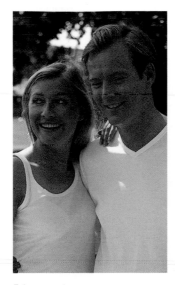

Fetus see **embryo**.

Follicle-stimulating hormone see **reproductive hormones**.

Genetic counselling Genetics is the science of heredity. Genetic counselling is offered to those couples who fail to conceive, who have repeated miscarriages or who have genetic disorders in their family medical histories.

GIFT (Gamete intra-Fallopian transfer) See pages 60–70.

ICSI (Intra-cytoplasm sperm injection) See pages 70–1.

In-vitro fertilization See pages 69–77.

Incompatibility Some women's bodies repel their partner's sperm. Some sperm is attacked by antibodies, which may be produced by either the man or woman. This biochemical incompatibility may be resolved by one of the methods of assisted fertility described in the chapter on delayed conception, pages 60–77.

IUI (Intrauterine insemination) See pages 60–77.

Laparoscopy A laparoscopy is a procedure in which a narrow tube with a telescopic eyepiece is inserted through a cut in the mother's abdomen. Light is transmitted along a cable within the tube and through the window at the top of the tube, enabling the surgeon to see into the abdomen and identify any problems or abnormalities that may be preventing conception. The procedure is carried out under general anaesthetic.

Luteinizing hormone see **reproductive hormones**.

Miscarriage This is the lay (non-medical) term for the spontaneous loss of a pregnancy. A large percentage of pregnancies are lost, often for no reason that can be determined, sometimes before the woman even knows that she is pregnant. The medical term for miscarriage is spontaneous abortion.

Motility Sperm gain the ability to move (known medically as motility) by means of a process that is not yet completely understood. Sperm are not able to swim. They are transported by muscular contractions through the man's reproductive system and, when they enter or are propelled into the woman's reproductive system, they continue to be transported.

Oestrogen This describes a number of hormones that are produced by the ovaries and the adrenal gland. During pregnancy, the placenta also produces oestrogen. The oestrogen hormones are responsible for the development of the female breasts and genitals at puberty and they also play a very important part in controlling the female menstrual cycle. During pregnancy, these hormones stimulate the growth of the uterus and breast tissue. See also **reproductive hormones**.

Pre-eclampsia This is the precursor to a very serious convulsive condition that occurs in pregnancy and is known as eclampsia. Pre-eclampsia is characterized by the development of high blood pressure, swelling (especially of the face, ankles, and wrists), and by the appearance of protein in the urine. Urgent referral to hospital is required.

Progesterone One of the female hormones, progesterone is produced by the corpus luteum in the ovary, to a lesser extent by the adrenal gland, and in pregnancy by the placenta. Progesterone is responsible for building up the endometrium in the uterus, which feeds the developing embryo during the early days of pregnancy. This hormone stimulates the growth of the mother-to-be's glandular, milk-producing tissue and helps smooth muscle to relax. See also **reproductive hormones**.

Reproductive hormones The menstrual cycle is controlled by the reproductive hormones, FSH (follicle-stimulating hormone) and LH (luteinizing hormone). These reproductive hormones are released by the brain and stimulate the ovaries to produce the female sex hormones, oestrogen and progesterone.

Sperm count This is the number of sperm in any one ejaculate of semen. A low sperm count is a well-known cause of infertility.

ZIFT (Zygote intra-Fallopian transfer) See pages 70–7.

Useful addresses and websites

UNITED KINGDOM
Foresight, The Association for the Promotion of Preconceptual Care
28 The Paddock
Godalming, Surrey GU7 1XD
tel: 01483 427839
www.foresight-preconception.org.uk

The Human Fertilisation and Embryology Authority
Paxton House
30 Artillery Lane, London E1 7LS
tel: 020 7377 5077
www.hfea.gov.uk/ForPatients

Infertility Network UK
Charter House
43 St Leonard's Road
Bexhill-on-Sea, East Sussex TN40 1JA
tel: 01424 732361   www.child.org.uk

Miscarriage Association
Clayton Hospital
Northgate, Wakefield
West Yorkshire WF1 3JS
tel: 01924 200799   www.the-ma.org.uk

National Childbirth Trust
Alexander House
Oldham Terrace
Acton, London W3 6NH
tel: 0870 4448707
breastfeeding support line: 0870 4448708
www.nctpregnancyandbabycare.com

Relate (relationship counselling)
Herbert Gray College
Little Church Street
Rugby, Warwickshire CV21 3AP
tel: 01788 573241
Helpline: 0845 1304010
www.relate.org.uk

Royal College of Obstetricians and Gynaecologists
27 Sussex Place, London NW1 4RG
tel: 020 7772 6200
www.rcog.org.uk

Complementary Therapies
The British Register of Complementary Practitioners (BRCP)
Institute for Complementary Medicine
PO Box 194
London SE16 7QZ
tel: 020 7237 5165
www.icmedicine.co.uk

ACUPUNCTURE
The British Acupuncture Council
63 Jeddo Road
London W12 9HQ
tel: 020 8735 0400
www.acupuncture.org.uk

ALEXANDER TECHNIQUE
The Society of Teachers of the Alexander Technique
1st Floor, Linton House
Highgate Entrance
39–51 Highgate Road, London NW5 1RS
tel: 0845 230 7828   www.stat.org.uk

AROMATHERAPY
The International Federation of Aromatherapists
182 Chiswick High Road
London W4 1PP
tel: 020 8742 2605   www.ifaroma.org

BACH FLOWER REMEDIES
Bach Centre
Mount Vernon, Sotwell, Wallingford,
Oxon OX10 0PZ   tel: 01491 834678
www.bachcentre.com

CHIROPRACTIC
General Chiropractic Council
44 Wicklow Street, London WC1X 9HL
Tel: 0207 713 5155   www.gcc-uk.org

HERBALISM
The National Institute of Medical Herbalists
56 Longbrook Street, Exeter EX4 6AH
tel: 01392 426022   www.nimh.org.uk

HOMEOPATHY
The British Homeopathic Association
Hahnemann House, 29 Park Street West,
Luton LU1 3BE
tel: 0870 4443950
www.trusthomeopathy.org

MASSAGE
The London College of Massage
5 Newman Passage, London W1T 1EH
tel: 020 7323 3574
www.massagelondon.com

MEDITATION
The School of Meditation
158 Holland Park Avenue
London W11 4UH   tel: 020 7603 6116
www.schoolofmeditation.org

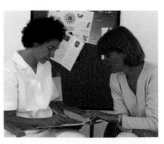

OSTEOPATHY
The General Osteopathic Council
Osteopathy House, 176 Tower Bridge Rd,
London SE1 3LU   tel: 020 7357 6655
www.osteopathy.org.uk

PILATES
The Body Control Pilates Association
7 Langley Street, London WC2H 9JA
www.bodycontrol.co.uk

REFLEXOLOGY
Association of Reflexologists
27 Old Gloucester Street
London WC1N 3XX
tel: 0870 5673320   www.aor.org.uk

YOGA
British Wheel of Yoga
25 Jermyn Street
Sleaford, Lincolnshire NG34 7RU
tel: 01529 306851   www.bwy.org.uk

UNITED STATES
The American College of Obstetricians and Gynecologists
409 12th Street NW
Washington DC 200024-2188
tel: 202 638 5577   www.acog.org

National Women's Health Network
514 10th Street NW
Washington DC 20004 tel: 202 347 1140
www.womenshealthnetwork.org

Resolve (fertility problems)
1310 Broadway
Somerville MA 02144-1779
tel: 617 623 0744   www.resolve.org

Complementary Therapies
American Holistic Medical Association
12101 Menaul Blvd., NE, Suite C
Albuquerque NM 87112 tel: 505 292 7788
www.holisticmedicine.org

ACUPUNCTURE
American Association of Oriental Medicine
5530 Wisconsin Avenue
Suite 1210, Chevy Chase MD 20815
tel: 301 941 1064   www.aaom.org

CHIROPRACTIC
American Chiropractic Association
1701 Clarendon Boulevard
Arlington VA 22209
tel: 800 986 4636   www.amerchiro.org

HERBALISM
American Herbalists Guild
1931 Gaddis Road, Canton GA 30115
tel: 770 751 6021
www.americanherbalistsguild.com

HOMEOPATHY

National Center for Homeopathy
801 North Fairfax Street
Suite 306, Alexandria VA 22314
tel: 703 548 7790
www.homeopathic.org

HYPNOTHERAPY

American Institute of Hypnotherapy
1805 E Garry Avenue
Suite 100, Santa Ana CA 92705
tel: 714 261 6400
www.aih.cc

MASSAGE

American Massage Therapy Association
1701 820 Davis Street, Suite 100,
Evanston IL 60201
tel: 847 864 0123
www.amtamassage.org

OSTEOPATHY

American Osteopathic Association
142 East Ontario Street
Chicago IL 60611
tel: 312 202 8000
www.osteopathic.org

REFLEXOLOGY

International Institute of Reflexology
PO Box 12642, St Petersburg FL 33733
tel: 813 343 4811
www.reflexology-usa.net

YOGA

International Association of Yoga Therapists
PO Box 426, Manton CA 96059
tel: 530 474 5700   www.yrec.org

CANADA

Infertility Network
160 Pickering Street, Toronto, Ontario
M4E 3J7   tel: 416 690 8015
www.infertilitynetwork.org

Canadian Women's Health Network
Suite 203, 419 Graham Avenue
Winnipeg, Manitoba R3C 0M3
tel: 204 942 5500   www.cwhn.ca

AUSTRALIA

Australian Complementary Health Association
247 Flinders Lane, Melbourne, Vic 3000
tel: (03) 9650 5327 www.diversity.org.au

Fertility Society of Australia
61 Danks Street
Port Melbourne
Vic 3207   tel: 03 9645 6349
www.fsa.au.com

Australian Women's Health Network
www.awhn.org.au

NEW ZEALAND

The New Zealand Health Information Network
PO Box 337, Christchurch 8015
tel: 03 980 4646   www.nzhealth.net.nz

New Zealand Infertility Society
PO Box 34151, Birkenhead
Auckland
tel: 0800 333 306
www.nzinfertility.org.nz

SOUTH AFRICA

www.childbirth.co.za
www.aotivebirth.co.za

African Health Anthology
www.nisc.co.za

Further reading and Acknowledgements

FURTHER READING

Belinda Barnes and Suzanne Gail Bradley/in association with Foresight, the Association for the Promotion of Preconceptual Care *Planning for a Healthy Baby* (Vermilion, London, 1994; Random House in Australia, New Zealand and South Africa)

Marilyn Glenville *Natural Solutions to Infertility* (Piatkus, London, 2000)

Doviel Hall and Françoise Barbira Freedman *Prenatal Yoga for Conception, Pregnancy and Birth* (Lorenz Books, London, 2002)

Harriet Griffey *How to Get Pregnant* (Bloomsbury, London, 1997)

Maggie Jones *Infertility: Modern Treatments and the Issues They Raise* (Piatkus, London, 1991)

Sally Keeble: *Conceiving Your Baby: How Medicine Can Help* (Cedar/Mandarin, London, 1995)

Dr Mary Ann Lumsden et al *Royal College of Obstetricians and Gynaecologists/ Complete Women's Health* (Thorsons, London, 2000)

Vivien Marx *The Semen Book* (Free Association Books, London, 2001)

Dr Ann Robinson *The Which? Guide to Women's Health* (Which? Books, London, 1999)

Sherman J Silber, MD *How to Get Pregnant with The New Technology* (Warner Books, USA, 1998)

Allan Templeton et al *Management of Infertility for the MRCOG and Beyond* (RCOG Press, London, 2000)

Professor Robert Winston, MB, BS, FRCOG *Getting Pregnant: The Complete Guide to Fertility and Infertility* (Pan, London, Sydney and Auckland, 1989)

Professor Robert Winston, MB, BS, FRCOG *Infertility: A Sympathetic Approach* (Martin Dunitz, London, 1986)

ACKNOWLEDGEMENTS

Anne Charlish:
I am grateful to Mr Donald Gibb, to Professor Gedis Grudzinskas and Patricia Roberts for their assistance over many years on the subjects of pregnancy and birth. I am grateful to Mr Malcolm Whitehead for his insights into the menopause and premature menopause. Lastly, I am greatly indebted to Professor Robert Winston for his tireless research and illuminating publications into the complex subject of fertility.

Publisher:
The Publishers are grateful to the following picture libraries for permission to reproduce the photographs listed below in this book (all those not listed below are © Anness Publishing Ltd):
t=top; b=bottom; c=centre; l=left; r=right

Science Photo Library:
p45 tl /BSIP, Chassenet; p60 /BSIP, HARDAS; p67 bl and br /James King-Holmes; p70 br /Alexander Tsiaras; p71 tl; Astier; p86 br /Mark Thomas

Corbis:
p43 bl /Larry Williams; p47 /Norbert Schaefer; p49 cr /Royalty-free; p53 tr /Royalty-free; p69 t Corbis only

The publishers would also like to thank:
MOT Models agency; Pregnant Pause Agency; the Warehouse studio (location setting); Bonieventure Bagalue for assisting photographer Alistair Hughes; Sue Duckworth for helping with props; Chris Bernstein for the index; Doriel Hall and Françoise Freedman for use of material on yoga, which we have adapted, mainly on pp56/7.

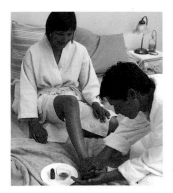

Index

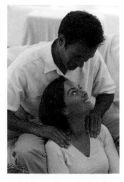

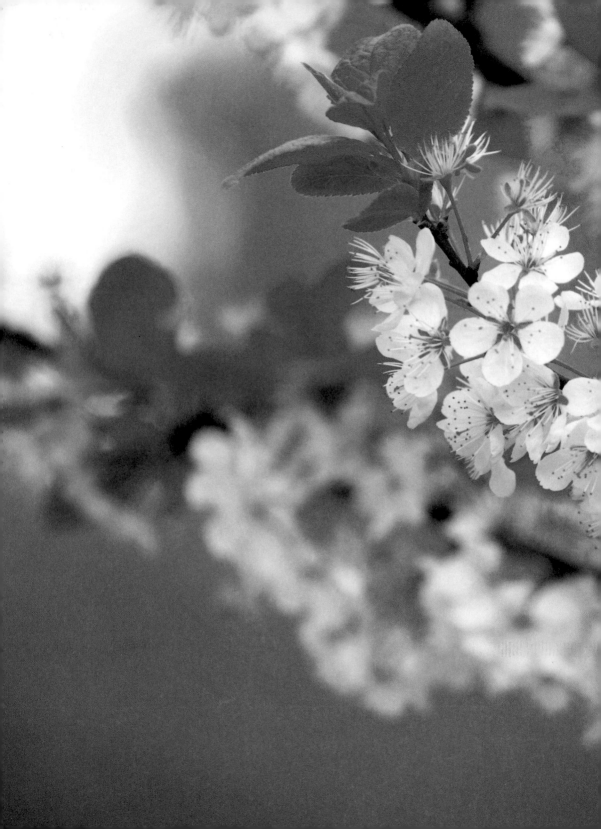